The Body's Map of Consciousness

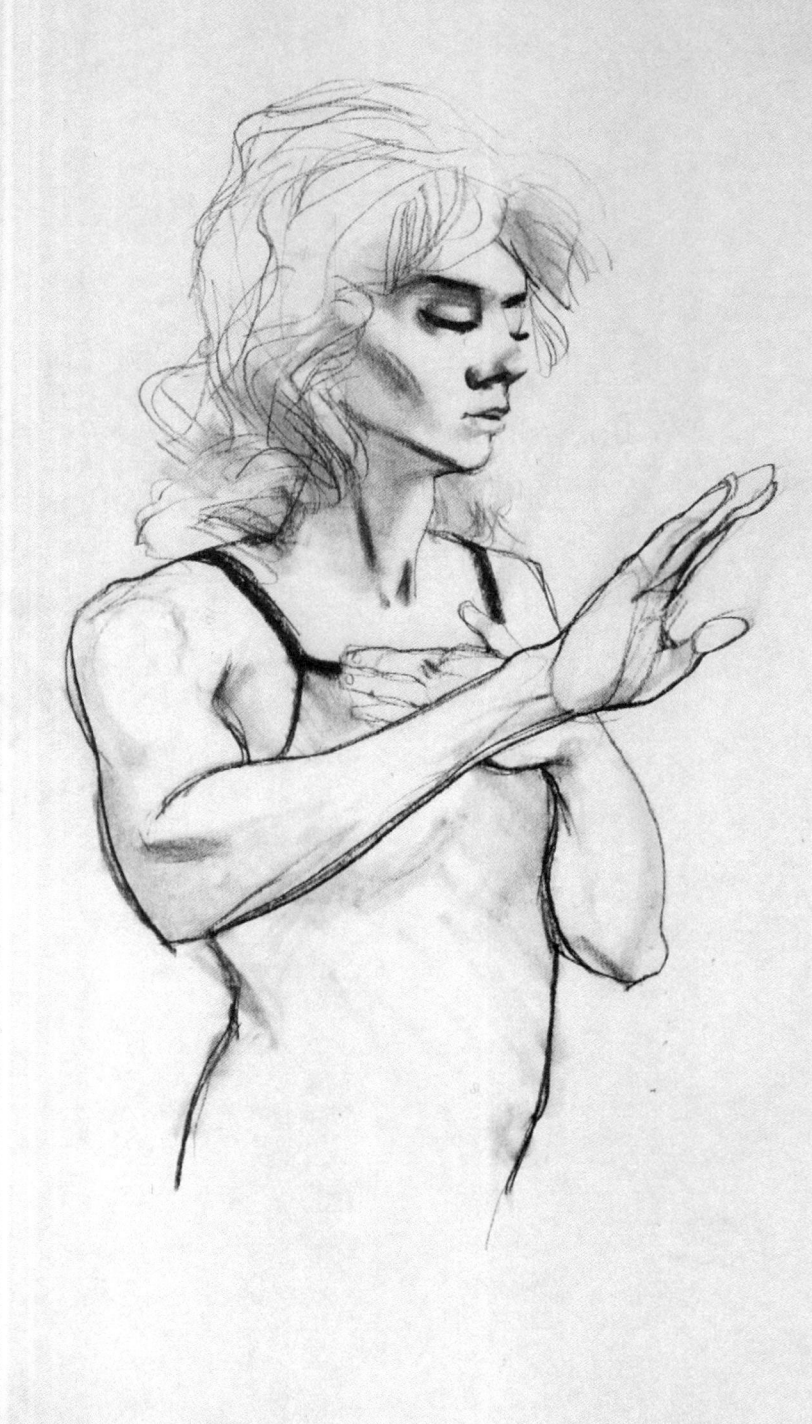

THE BODY'S MAP
of CONSCIOUSNESS

VOLUME 1: *Movement*

Lansing Barrett Gresham   Julie J. Nichols
Illustrations by Ken Macklin

© 2002 Lansing Barrett Gresham and Julie J. Nichols. All rights reserved.

Cover art and Illustrations © 2002 Ken Macklin. No drawing from this book may be reproduced without permission of the artist.

Book Design © 2002 sethtaylor.com

ISBN 1-893969-01-0

Integrated Awareness® and The Body's Map of Consciousness® are registered to Lansing Barrett Gresham.

For further information about IA workshops, events, or teachers near you, visit www.inawareness.com or call NoneTooSoon Publishing (801.363.1747) or Touchstone (707.795.4399).

By the same authors:

*Ask Anything, and Your Body Will Answer:
A Personal Journey Through Integrated Awareness*

Lansing's Acknowledgments

To: the true author of this book,
Julie J. Nichols, without whom even
the first word would still be
unwritten

My first teachers, my parents Charlene and Robert

My examples Skip & Toni, Nicki and Ron

My once-upon-a-time comrades, Bob and Jim, Will and Allan

My heartbreaks, Barbara & Laurel & Kathryn

My professional models: June & Michael & Moshe' & John, & Jean-Pierre

My allies Barbara Jean & Dale & Randy & Ellen; Barbara & Michael, Anne & Toby, Dean & Deb, Peter & Collette;

Those beloved souls whose relation is beyond my ability to categorize

The thousands of students and colleagues who have given so much meaning to my life;

To my inspirations for the future
SAM AND MOLLIE AND JACK

And to Deborah
who held my feet to the karmic fire
when my courage alone
was not enough

MY GRATITUDE IN EVERY LIFE.

Julie's Acknowledgments

The material described and defined in *The Body's Map of Consciousness* has been developed over decades and is still in process. However, in the three years since Lansing first told me he wanted this book to be written, I have been lovingly encouraged, supported, and put up with by family members, friends, and the Integrated Awareness community, and for this I am truly grateful.

My husband Jeff (Nick) and our children have graciously deferred to me when I needed time, space, travel, or the household computer. Their love and humor are central to my life.

My parents, Clyde and Carol Juchau, have been financially supportive and always interested. My brother Dan Juchau of San Jose, California, has lent transportation and given much-needed advice many times. My sister Jan Argyle has been a source of laughter and down-to-earth moral support. My colleagues and students in the Department of English and Literature at Utah Valley State College in Orem, Utah, have been humane and good-natured while I juggled work on this project with work related to them. My clients and friends at 893 South McClelland have been full of light and laughter. To all of you, thanks.

In Utah, Diana West, Alison Craig, and PJ Hair read and astutely commented on versions of the manuscript. I am grateful to those in California who did the same: Anne Woodhead, Barbara Jean Veronda, Ellen Rayner, Linda Tumey, and Randy Post. Nationwide, Heidi McGuire, Marcelyn Smith (Watson), Beryl Feinglass, Sue Holmes, Michelle Smith, Catherine Barritt, fellow students in the Course in Self-Trust at Touchstone, and to a lesser degree other members of the IA community housed, fed, transported, communicated with, applauded, and otherwise sustained me warmly and kindly. To them, and particularly to those who contributed anecdotes to this volume—Ellen, Rondi Boyer, and Kathleen Marquardt—a special thanks.

Jan Worseley Cendese has been a wonderful colleague and friend in Salt Lake City. Ellen Rayner has been unflagging in her physical, emotional, and spiritual support for this project; she is amazing. For their help in designing and printing the book, I am indebted to Seth Taylor and everyone at Press Publishing. For her beautiful modeling for the cover, I am in awe of Claudia Larson. For his cheerful, prompt, highly pleasing work as illustrator, I cannot praise Ken Macklin enough.

Finally, it has to be acknowledged that Lansing is the *author* of this book. He dictated, explained, demonstrated, and explored every word and process here, over hours and hours of telephone and face-to-face interaction. As the *writer,* I am indebted to him for his patient and painstaking revisions. This book is meant to reflect accurately his experiences and teaching; I am to blame for any deviation from his design. He has also contributed a *great* deal of emotional and financial support for the project. Throughout, there has been synergy requiring the enthusiastic effort of both of us.

I thank our many teachers and forerunners, too, for bringing so much light to the human condition—its largeness, its multidimensionality, its so-often-ignored-or-forgotten possibility. The form Lansing has brought to this material—which we've only begun to describe here (looking forward to Volumes 2 and 3!)—always inspires me. Lansing's influence as teacher and ally uplifts and comforts me very nearly one hundred percent of the time.

TABLE OF CONTENTS

I. Introduction: If You've Ever Thought, "There Must Be More To Life…"—You're Right! 01
II. Ingrams 11
III. Inner/Outer/Inter-Space 17
   The function in consciousness of spatial components of the body's map
IV. You Are Designed For Movement 23
V. Movement Teams and Planar Relationships 27
VI. Posture 35
   An exploration of standing posture
VII. Barriers: Moving and Not 41
   Movement process: Exploring with the arms
VIII. Floor Work 51
   Floor Process: Discovery and resolution of an emotional barrier.
IX. Defining a Matrix: Your Rules are Your Patterns 57
X. Shame and Deliverance 59
   The shame matrix and the matrix for acceptance
XI. Integrated Awareness 69
   Floor Process: Integrating the physical, emotional, and mental bodies

Afterword 87

Appendix A Two movement processes 89
   A.1. Finding a third choice
   A.2. Recruiting and integrating parts of yourself

Appendix B. Advanced Movement Teams 97

CHAPTER I

Introduction: If you've ever thought, "There must be more to life..."—you're right!

Integrated Awareness® is an innately human set of skills for healing and wholeness through *movement, touch,* and *change in consciousness*. One of its primary tools is a unique set of descriptions we call The Body's Map of Consciousness®. Many body mapping systems exist. This one, empirically developed over three decades of direct experience and observation of tens of thousands of people, is *built into* you, and we believe that it is *designed* to be explored and verified by anyone with the willingness and curiosity to do so.

Its fundamental principle is that *every site on or in your physical structure* is *predisposed to resonate with* one or more *specific other levels of consciousness*—other body sites, emotions, thought patterns, and many other aspects of yourself. Your physical movements (or lack thereof) literally embody these resonances. Exploration of movement patterns can increase awareness of limiting rules and inhibitions, which can then lead to the possibility of choosing to move differently—to invite different behaviors, different thought patterns, different ways to respond to life's experiences much more in keeping with your happiness and health.

How does this work?

Earth reality gives us this basic design: Time runs one way. Life forms become increasingly complex. Gravity pulls us toward the planet's core. All beings have gender. All are born and will die. All these (and other) elements exist in human experience to varying degrees of health and harmony *depending primarily on whether we are willing for energy to move or not.* In other words, health and harmony are a function of *choice*.

Everything on this planet, and indeed the planet itself, is energy, motion, and the consciousness that drives it. Current physics studies suggest that energy is never still. Energy is always in motion, and every

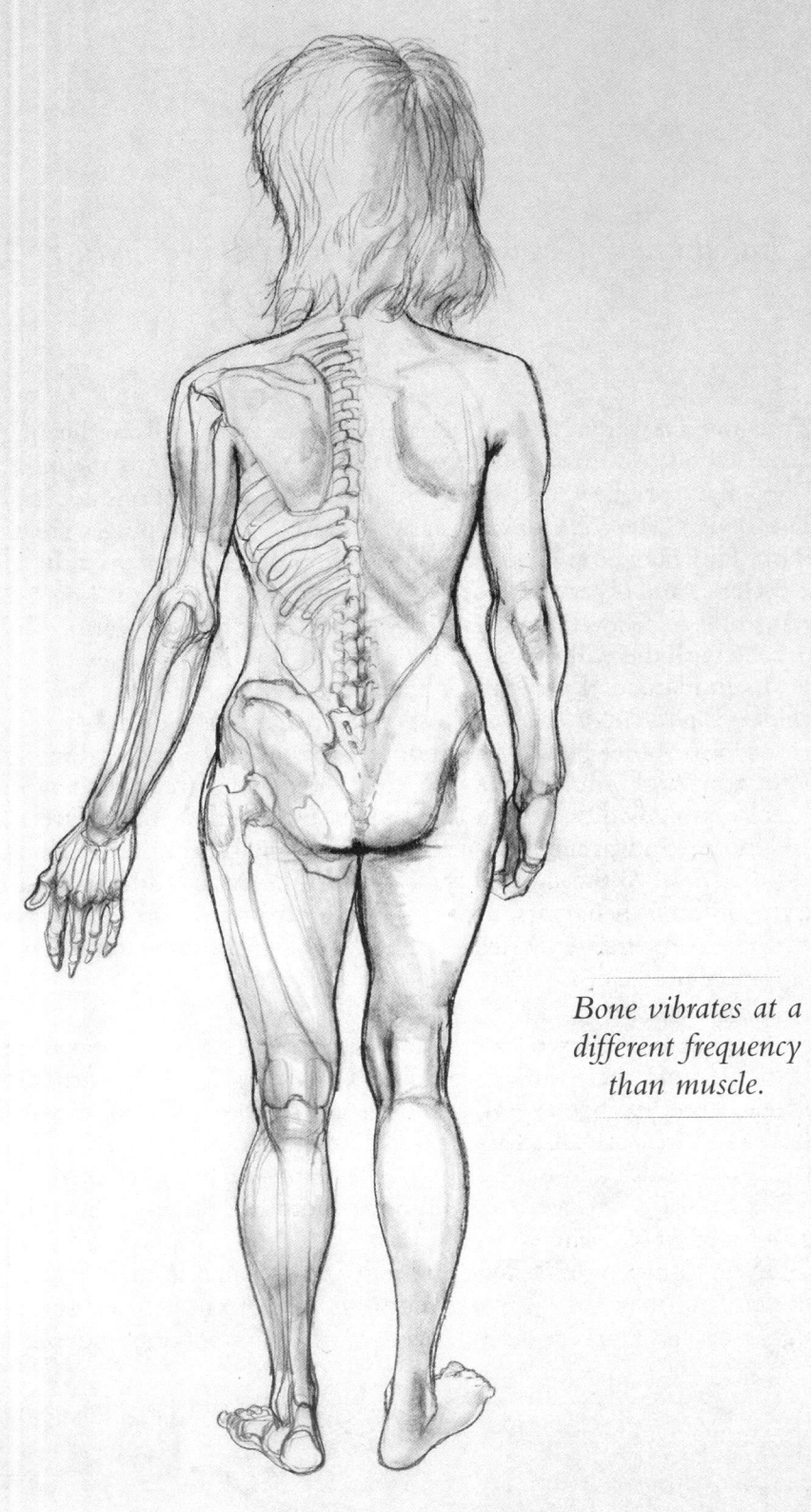

Bone vibrates at a different frequency than muscle.

distinguishable thing on earth—including every distinct body site and part—has its own base vibrational note. Its fundamental atomic state is distinct from that of even the most nearby distinct location or feature.

This underlying quality of vibration predisposes it to respond more to some vibrations and less to others. Those responses can be amplifying, harmonic, dissonant, or neutralizing. Think of a stringed instrument. When you pluck an A string, for example, another instrument's A string will vibrate faintly in response. If the second instrument's A string is plucked intentionally along with the first, the note is amplified, increased, louder, stronger. If a finger is placed on a certain site on the fingerboard, you may hear a pleasing (harmonic) combination of tones or a not-so-pleasing one (dissonant). Now think of a food you like and consider how the taste is amplified by certain other foods, complemented by yet others, and canceled out by yet others. And think of the color wheel, with tones that can complement each other or clash.

The principle is the same, though the medium—the form of the energy whose vibrational note is being responded to—is different. When we speak of consciousness, movement and energy interacting with each other, we are describing exactly these same universal earthly principles of vibration, harmony and disharmony, resonance and dissonance.

To bring this to the realm of your human system, it can be felt that bone vibrates—moves—at a different frequency than fluid. Nerves vibrate differently from connective tissue. Thoughts operate at a different level, and within a different vibrational spectrum, than do emotions. Just as in music, different octaves have the same notes such that some clash, some blend, and some complement without blending or clashing, so, too, different tissues, thoughts and feelings, also blend, clash, or contrast for highlight and emphasis.

In other words, emotions have intrinsic harmonic relation to particular body sites, mental constructs and all other simple or complex aspects of human existence. This is how the body's map works.

> Ellen's first experience of Integrated Awareness® was at an evening introductory workshop. She says, "Admittedly I was skeptical and I agreed to go only to satisfy the constant urgings of a good friend. One of the first instructions given was to shut our eyes and internally assess the shape and

size of our eye sockets. Seemed like a rather strange thing to do. I was surprised to discover, though, that if I paid close attention I could actually sense differences between my two eyes.

"We were told the left side of the body resonates with female essence, and the right with male. We were asked to cover the eye corresponding to our own gender with the hand on the same side, and then the eye associated with the other gender with the hand that we had just used. Again, curiosity got the best of me, and I went along with the instruction, only to discover sensations and differences that I had no idea existed.

"Then came the instruction to do the same process with the other hand (in my case, the right hand, the one associated with male). I was totally stunned when I covered my left eye with my right hand. Everything went dark, there was absolutely no sensation or awareness of self in this configuration! I immediately raised my hand and asked, 'How could this be?'

"The instructor's gentle answer was to ask if I was surprised that I disappear and completely devalue myself *when I am observed as female from my recordings and projections of male perspective.* Bingo. I was captivated. This was the beginning of self-discovery and exploration in Integrated Awareness that ultimately changed my life."

The human body is such an extraordinarily intricate set of overlapping, interwoven and even competing frequencies that sorting through them can feel overwhelming. Yet this stunningly complex reality is exactly the background and foundation upon which every human infant must build its construct of reality. And everyone has multiple capacities for perceiving these resonances at all times.

It begins with simply acknowledging what you feel. "Yes, I feel good (fluid, easy, congruent, available in a relaxed but alert way)." "No, things don't feel right (they feel dissonant)." "Something's off (not resonant with you or with other factors in the environment)."

Or "This is miraculous (uncommonly resonant—to the point of oneness and pure good feeling)..."

You're in business, striding your way from meeting to meeting, office to office. On any given day you encounter dozens of people of all shapes and attitudes. You begin to note with increasing puzzlement the pulled-down mouths, drawn-up shoulders, puckered foreheads, and rigid stances of your colleagues. Young retailers whose eyes won't meet yours...middle-aged vendors with shoulders hunched up around their ears walking as if their hips and ankles hurt... long-time CEO's gazing absently with eyebrows drawn together and head tipped slightly back or to one side as if disconnected from the rest of their body. Body types and postures reflect as many emotional states and degrees of presence as there are people.

You're a teacher. You feel the effort it is to sit still in those chairs and rows of desks, the lethargy of the students after lunch, their agitation at the end of the day. You're acutely conscious of the only-partial success with which you seem to transfer information. There's more to learning than linear words and two-dimensional paper, and more to the students than mental constructs. What exactly is it?

You're an artist, a sculptor, a cook, a writer, an equestrian. You've always been acutely aware of the aesthetics of your work, the relationships of tools, instruments, and raw materials to your own skills and intentions. You take delight in the creations of fellow artists. You also feel a need for a way to talk about "the zone," "beauty," even "excellence" that transcends either mere technique or academic criticism, to acknowledge more explicitly and invite more consistently the mysterious combination of awarenesses that produces success through you. You sense a force that enlarges you with one pure intent, and it fills you with gratitude. What is it?

You're a health caregiver. Saddened on the one hand by the apparent inability of some people to heal and shocked by the rise in the incidence of diseases, and aware, on the other hand, of the confusing power of placebo and of numerous spontaneous healings of the untreatable, you have grown certain that there's more to healing than drugs or surgery can offer. There must be something else to help account for what happens in our physical bodies all the time.

Belonging to one of the above categories or not, you still feel yourself to be "an ordinary person."

International politics, finance, speculative fiction and somber nonfiction, ancient and not-so-ancient predictions from Tibetan, Hindi, Aztec, Amarind, and even Protestant traditions, all tell us that we may have as little as twenty years in which to effect a fundamental alteration in the base level of consciousness on the planet. We hold the tools for our own evolution in myriad forms. We engineer our own genetics, make or break economic systems, distribute resources to or withhold them from those who need them. We can annihilate whole cultures or countries or continents with the push of a button (or with a box-cutter and a firm resolve to die for a cause). It almost seems to you as if circumstances in our polarized, conflict-ridden culture are moving toward a climax of life-and-death proportions.

If it has become impossible for you not to notice in the faces, postures and behaviors of your friends and family the expressions of a vast array of seemingly uncontrollable conditions, from illness and emotional drought to the very heights of wellness and inspiration—then it's likely you too are thinking, "There's more to life than most systems will acknowledge! There must be more! And if there is—there *should* be more to *me*!"

If you've thought these things, perhaps you have intuited Integrated Awareness® and The Body's Map of Consciousness®.

What are *levels of consciousness*? You're actually quite familiar with this concept. *Bodies,* as in "I can tell that my physical and emotional bodies are interdependent because when I'm sad, I cry." *Parts,* as in "there's a part of her that wants to marry, and another part that wants to remain single." *States,* as in "my mental state was quite confused." *Vibrations,* as in "he gave off a loving vibration." *Field,* as in "if we let that degree of conflict into the field, we may never reach resolution."

A "level of consciousness" in this context isn't an esoteric or etheric construct you have to be psychic to experience. As you move naturally from one aspect of your life to another, you change the dominance and relative proportions of awareness through which you view and filter your experiences. Sometimes you focus on the physical level, sometimes on the emotional, sometimes on the mental.

The magnificent truth related to these levels of consciousness is that all of them are at work all the time. Even when you don't realize it, because you are focusing on only one or another aspect of any given situation, you're still busy registering physical, emotional, and mental responses to stimuli all the time—because you are *built* to do so.

A simple analogy can be found in the study of genetics. It's commonly held that each gene, and many gene combinations on your particular DNA map predispose you to a huge variety of tendencies, forms, and experiences, from the color of your eyes to your susceptibility to emotional and physical illnesses and even your manner of death. You have, in potential, the capacity for hundreds, if not an infinite number, of possibilities in the way your life plays itself out. Because many factors—some of them internal and some external—determine which of these potentials are activated, you express only a small part of those tendencies at any one time and, indeed, in any one *lifetime*. Nevertheless, the potential for all of them exists all the time, throughout your life.

In exactly the same way, every site on your entire physical structure that's distinct from any other site—your left first index knuckle, the lateral collateral ligament of your right knee, your duodenum, your third cervical vertebra—has a distinct association with one or more specific other levels of consciousness, which are all continuously operating. And from the moment of your conception, any and all of these may be associated in your consciousness with any of a huge number of external factors as well.

INTRODUCTION

You carry in your physical body the potential for an infinite variety of stress and movement patterns, inhibitions and limitations, which depend for activation in very specific ways on stimulus and response. The implications are rather staggering.

First, your physical structure as it is today is a reliable record of all aspects of all your levels of consciousness, from your first moment to now. The postures and movement patterns of your body reflect the areas in your life where you have internalized contradictions and conflicts; where you have unconsciously assigned eternal associations to elements that are in reality only temporarily or even only seemingly related; or where you have imposed on yourself rules about not moving or not behaving in any particular way in response to any particular experience.

Second, you can choose to change. You can develop the kinesthetic and proprioceptive perceptual skill to allow you to consciously recognize differing qualities of movement, the presence or absence of movement in different places in your body. With the body's map you can acknowledge the origin or content of those variations and patterns in movement. And you can choose to make the movements you now refuse and improve the quality of the movements you now make with difficulty. No more than that—and the courage to explore—is required.

Every map—any map—describes sites, functions, and patterns against a background. The body's map of consciousness is *built into you* as a primary source of data as you seek to explore your purposes on earth. The "background" is your entire consciousness. The "sites" are distinct locations on or in your physical structure. The many kinds of vibrational associations within your entire system are the "functions" in the body's map of consciousness. And the "patterns" are discernible links between sites and functions.

Indeed, the body's map is complex and wonderful. But it is not mysterious. In the first chapters we present foundational information:

- **Touch, movement,** and **change of consciousness** as fundamental tools of Integrated Awareness® and The Body's Map®;
- the existence of many associational patterns within you, including **ingrams**;
- the **spatial components** of the body's map;
- an explanation of the reasons that **position** and **movement** are

the best mirrors of your body's adaptations and behaviors; and
- explanations of directional and allied components of movement (**movement teams** and **planar relationships**).

The rest of the chapters apply and extend the above information, inviting you to discover within yourself the associations in consciousness between many spatial and movement aspects of your physical structure, and your other levels of consciousness. These will not be exactly the same for everyone. Read slowly. Practice gently. No faster than you feel able to proceed, explore:
- a **standing** posture
- relatively simple **movements** and movement prohibitions (**barriers**)
- a definition and example of a multi-level set of associations (**matrix**)
- several **movement processes** to allow you to experience for yourself the body's map's complexity and the magnitude of data available, which can lead directly to an expanded sense of all that you really are. Exploring the body's map can radically shift (and may finally end) any idea of compartmentalization—of you; of the parts of your life; of your sense of your relation to all other lives; and of souls.

Your body's map is personal and innate. You will not learn it, ultimately, from a book, or from any external source. IA classes consistently incorporate movement processes; IA is as much a way of learning as it is a body of knowledge—you, in fact, are literally a body of knowledge, which the body's map assists you to remember. There are great advantages in seeking the direction of a teacher to guide your explorations in the beginning and periodically, and we encourage you to do so. Many IA teachers throughout the United States are familiar with the processes in this book and are pledged to support and assist you.

In a classroom atmosphere or alone, it is essential for an optimum experience that you feel safe from the possibility of unexpected interruption. Allow for privacy. Remove or turn off your phone. Be sure the environment contains no obstacles to movement, and that you have the physical support you may need to move from the floor to a standing position, or any other kind of physical support necessary for you personally. Move slowly and gently. Let there be time afterward for solitude; invite space and time to process the information—ultimately sacred—which the experience reveals.

The symbol 👤 invites you to follow these steps:

- First, read the instructions all the way through.
- Then, if they are lengthy, record them on a tape player, leaving a minute or more of silence for each long space in the text.
- Play the recording back for yourself.
- Whether the instructions are short or long, close your eyes and go inside to make the observations asked of you. It may help if you are in a quiet, comfortable place by yourself.
- Alternatively, have a trusted friend read the instructions to you.

Following these steps will facilitate explorations.

The human physical structure is designed as a built-in database of stored information about behavior and its relation to emotional, mental, and other states. Through expanded awareness of the associations between physical structure and other levels of consciousness, any of us may begin to free ourselves from old habits, choose new behaviors, and discover a more satisfying, happier life.

CHAPTER II

Ingrams

In any moment, your *physical body* is in an arrangement, a posture or a movement—is doing some things and not others. In that same moment, your *brain chemistry* is framing some patterns and not others. Your *energy* is high or low, tensed or open. Your *emotions* are engaged. Your *mind* is working as fast as it can to make sense of it all.

The nervous system isn't wasteful. Early learning is by association, not by cause and effect. An infant doesn't conceive an origin for all those sensations she experiences! Nevertheless, the nervous system records all those associations for the infant. It remembers everything perceived in moments of joy or stress, taking note of and binding together every feeling, thought, and posture or movement that occur together.

> On a rainy February morning in a suburb of Seattle, in a yellow kitchen smelling of pancakes, a child seated in a high chair drops and breaks a glass of orange juice. His mother (whose favorite aunt died last week) cries out with peculiar intensity, and a dog barks and knocks the high chair over so that the child is flung face down on the floor.
>
> Without the child's conscious mental activity, all factors in the experience (including some we probably haven't even recognized!) become associated in that child's system with each other. Every time any one of these components comes up in his experience—rain, a barking dog, a glass of orange juice, the spilling of liquid, the sharp cry of a sad woman, a yellow interior, the odor of pancakes, the sensation of falling face down—all of them resonate to various degrees for him.
>
> Not only that, but over time he begins to assign cause to

these associations: drinking orange juice in a yellow kitchen will bring on the vibration, if not the occurrence, of spillage (whether it's liquid or a falling body). Or if a dog is brought inside, he expects something to smell of breakfast on a rainy day.

The older person who develops from the child in this example may have forgotten or may have only faint memories of the experience that ties those things together for him—but they *are* so tied. Unless he becomes aware of them and chooses to change them, his physical body continues to produce minute movements toward postures and activities that reflect his response to the associations recorded in his neurological system by this experience—movements which affect his posture and habits in myriad unacknowledged ways.

We call these associations *ingrams*—basic components of your "inner grammar." They are sets of correlated physical postures, brain patterns, energetic frequencies and emotional and mental constructs *which continue to occur together* for you *unless you choose consciously to disentangle them.*

Ingrams generally form before the age of three. From their caregivers and culture, very young children learn which behaviors are acceptable and which are not, which feel "okay" and which do not. As habits of behavior (or of avoidance) are developed, other choices are eliminated. For purposes of sheer survival, children prioritize all the correlated data bits associated with their experiences. It becomes necessary to (mostly) ignore, inhibit, dissociate from or deny the awareness that *many* kinds of activity are going on all the time in relation to particular body sites, movements, and postures.

By age five, associational patterns no longer receive full, integrated awareness; only particular ones valued by the culture or associated with positive or survival-assuring sensations are kept in awareness. And by adulthood, even less attention is paid to the possibility of other, alternative patterns or their implications. Because the habits are so ingrained by adulthood, even less information is available about the *reasons* for habits of behavior—or about the possibilities for new, spontaneous, often more appropriate and desirable behavior. Fewer choices are perceived.

It is essential to remember two things about ingrams. First, all of the components of an ingram are *associated* with one another in your awareness, whether consciously or not. (You don't have to be conscious of your genes for them to operate, either!) And second, as time passes, they become mistakenly projected as *causes*, each for all the others. The body's map of consciousness offers information to increase awareness of the components of these forgotten associations and the movement patterns that go with them, and to release you from the often-unrecognized immobilities and incapacities that go with them.

No part of the system is associated with only one thing. That this is embodied in the physical structure is illustrated by another example. Nearly all humans carry their heads tilted somewhat to one side or the other. If you put a ball on a stick and tilt the ball to one side, it's harder to carry the ball than if it's balanced on top of the stick. Gravity never cuts slack. In the same way, balancing your suitcase overhead is actually slightly easier than carrying it out to the side.

Now, tilting your head in one direction develops a habitual attitude and expression of self-image and point of view—literally, your physically-oriented perspective toward the world. This positioning of one part of your physical structure unbalances, creates asymmetry in, a host of other parts of you: the arteries and veins, the nerves, connective tissue, vertebrae, and muscles. Essentially, the functional range of all the body parts on one side become unequal to that on the other. In the standing position, this radiates downward such that the neck and shoulders are affected, as are the back, spine, arms, and visceral organs. If you follow this asymmetry down to the toes and the bottoms of the feet, you can perceive that all are different on the two sides. They change and adapt to the habit of carriage associated with your head tilt.

To test this, stand at the mirror, hold your head slightly to one side for five minutes and hold it to the other for five minutes. You will have no remaining doubt that your body has adapted to one of them. Holding your head tilted to the non-habitual side, you may find even two minutes difficult!

This is a relatively simple mechanical variation of a single body component. Each of those adapted parts of your physical structure below the head carries with it responsibilities of its own, necessary for your survival. It also carries emotional, mental, energetic, historical, temporal, genetic, and spiritual priorities in relation to which it is already individually hypersensitive. How the head tilts will reflect, maintain, and influence all of them.

You're made for *movement*. All living things move. Humans are designed to move with fluidity and grace. But restrictions begin to be placed on movement potential even within the womb. After birth, movements are inhibited or even blocked in highly specific ways, as we create and repeatedly enact our internal rules against behaviors which require certain movements. As you explore, it is possible to discover a completely personal and reliable record of your adaptations. It is just as possible to discover opportunities to release outdated "thou shalts" and "thou shalt nots." New behaviors can then be generated by restoring movement where there was none, by changing or softening the barriers erected by rules learned early in life, and by liberating other parts of yourself which you'd like to embrace.

Touch is the most direct sense, the one least blocked by the need for verbal interpretation. In infancy, touch is a person's most important way of receiving information. Touch transmits to the infant information about the caregiver's conscious and unconscious attitudes, and that information evolves into unquestioned components of self worth and the meaning of life. So touch is foundational to all subsequent values. Yet its non-linear, non-verbal nature tends to leave the significance of touch ignored by the intellectual and socialized self. A trained and sensitive toucher can remind you of many forgotten aspects of your own nature. Conscious, present touch can directly assist any of us in the process of becoming whole. Given the willingness and presence of the toucher *and* the one touched, it can allow us to reframe those associations from early infant handling.

A client of Kathleen's longed for a mother who had truly seen her, heard her, loved her for who she was. Unfortunately, her mother died before they could resolve their early difficulties. During a table session of IA, with her hands on her client's fully clothed body, Kathleen invited an updated, more mature presence of Mother into the client's infant body memories, allowing her to feel and grieve. The client chose to shift her perspective. "I didn't allow her to see me; I started adapting so soon she couldn't know how I was hurting. I didn't let her know me." Tears flowed, and a sense of forgiveness and understanding flowered. This session encouraged a new awareness of personal responsibility through touch.

Touch directly contacts physical structures and can influence movement. But it also affects the movement of energies within and around your body. We will address the touch component of Integrated Awareness® in our second volume, where we discuss the energy field more thoroughly, as well as brain patterns and the dimension of time.

Ultimately, exploring the body's map gives you the ability to *change your state or level of consciousness at will,* and to address many "higher" or more subtle vibratory frequencies. You know that you have felt "good vibes" and "bad vibes." You have intuited success and identified beauty; you've experienced what feels like chaos internally; and you've been transported to a sense of harmony. Everyone has. All of these are changes in state of consciousness. This will be the focus of the third volume. *Choosing* the priority of states or levels of consciousness allows a shift in focus to aspects of the self from which new decisions of movement and behavior can be made that may literally re-create your life. *You can respond consciously in the direction of harmony,* rather than react away from disharmony. You can literally *be more present,* be more yourself.

Just as no part of you is truly separate from other parts of you, so the body's map of consciousness is finally not separable into "movement," "touch," or "change in consciousness." Movement is not by any means the *simplest* component of Integrated Awareness. However, we consider movement to be a basic component of the body's map of consciousness upon which all others build. Ultimately, exploring your structure and movement patterns can integrate awareness of all parts of you—all levels of consciousness, physically, emotionally, mentally, spiritually, and many other aspects of yourself which you intuit to be real but which you may have lost sight of for a time, and which you long to restore to full consciousness because your life can be richer, happier, more wonderful in every way.

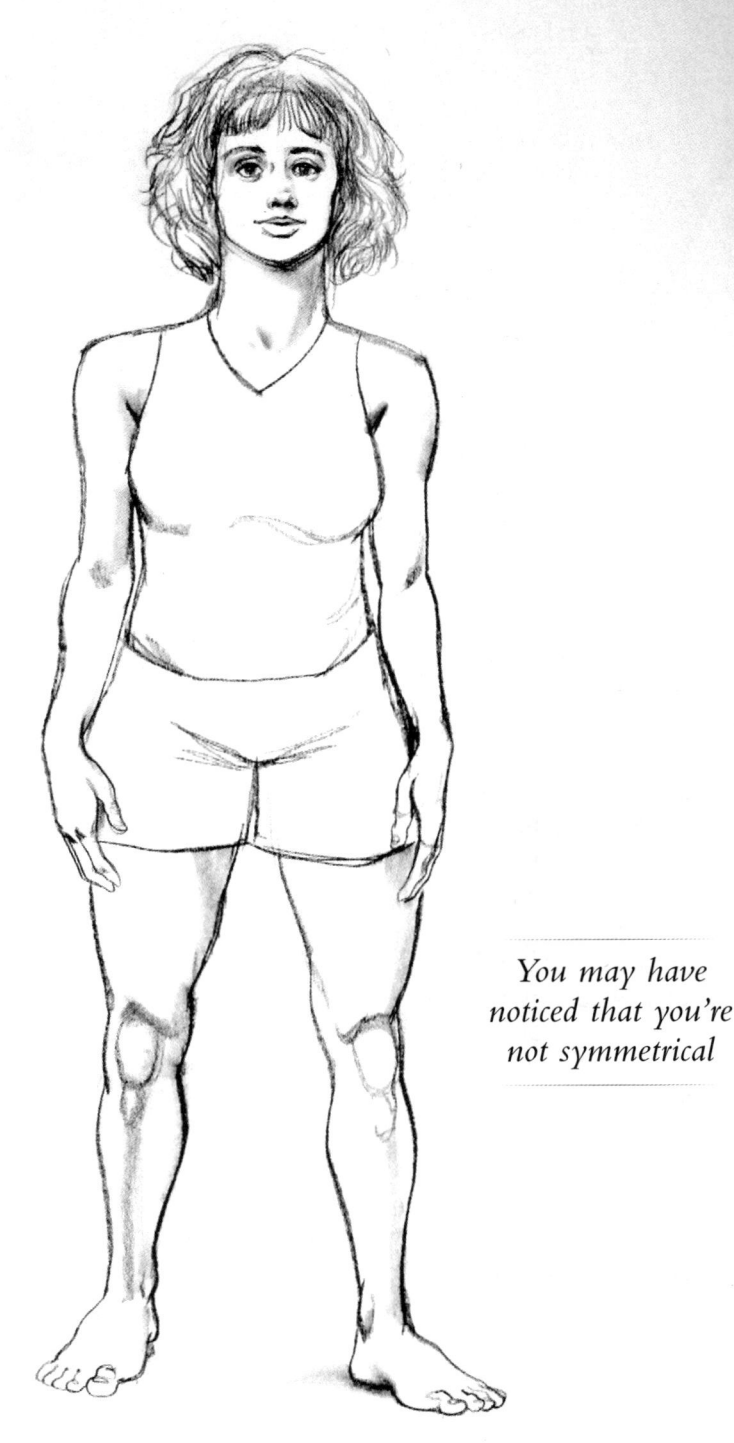

You may have noticed that you're not symmetrical

CHAPTER III

Inner- / Outer- / Inter-Space

There are a great many levels of consciousness. Three of the most commonly emphasized in American culture and therefore emphasized in this volume are the physical, the emotional, and the mental. Certain correlations among these have been consistently found to be true, whether exploration is through movement or touch. So we begin with fundamental spatial background components of the body's map—right/left, front/back, up/down, and core/periphery—and introduce the consistent correlations (or functions in consciousness) of each.

Right and left.
You may have noticed that you're not symmetrical. One eye is smaller than the other. One arm swings more freely than the other when you walk. The toes on one foot are shaped differently than those on the other. All of this is *associated with* (not caused by) experiences of, attitudes toward, and learned behaviors focusing on the two genders. Though you are one gender, you have interacted with both. And you feel, believe, and behave differently toward one than toward the other. The left side of the body embraces the entire composite with which female principle is manifested, and the right side is associated with male.

> Which hand is more clenched?
> Which arm is held when you walk?
> On which side of your body do you tend to sustain more illnesses or injuries? Which gender do you find yourself judging more or fearing more?

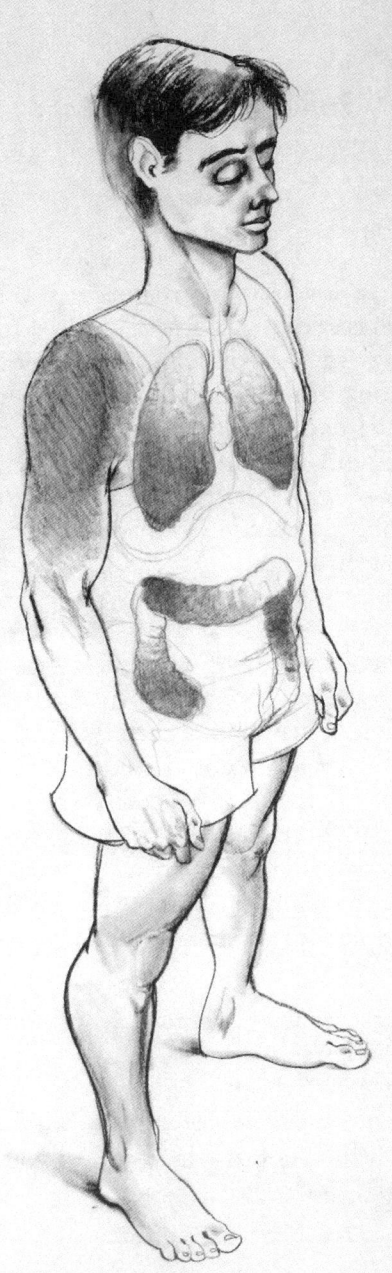

The closer a site or force or movement is to the beginning or the bottom—the first part of the colon, the bottom of the lung—the greater the probability that the important other levels became activated earlier.

Front and back.
The more to the front and (if exterior) easily seen a body site—your face, your palms, your kneecaps—the more the associated levels of consciousness are known to, active within, and influential over, the *strategies* of your conscious waking self. The more to the back or posterior, and the less often or less easily seen that part is—the base of your skull, the small of your back, the bend of your knee—the more the associated levels of consciousness exert their influence in ways you may not be so aware of in your waking life, because they have become part of the basic *construct* of your personality. This has been observed to be true not only for the front or back of your body generally, but also for the anterior or posterior aspect of any distinguishable body component or organ—lung, arm, etc.

> When you're sitting "upright," does your head tilt forward or back slightly (or a lot)? Do your physical aches and pains take you by surprise, or do you see them coming? What aspects of your life do you hide from yourself?

Bottom (or beginning) and top (or end).
The closer a site or force or movement is to what might be anatomically described as the beginning, or the bottom, of any part of your structure—the soles of the feet, the first part of the colon, the bottom of the lung—the greater the probability that the important other levels of consciousness associated with that site became activated *earlier* in your life. (Think of a painting—the earliest layers are laid down first.) The nearer the end or the top of any component the activity is, the more likely the associated levels are to have become important more recently or currently.

> What do you consider the origins of your issues? How far back in time can you go in waking memory? In feeling? In dreams or meditation? Allow yourself to trace any organ or body part to its "beginning." See what you discover.

SPATIAL COMPONENTS

Core and periphery.
The more toward the core of the body a location, a movement, a force, the more you associate it directly with yourself. The further to the periphery of the body, the more you associate it with your interactions with others.

To make it easier to orient all this information to your personal life circumstances, here is an example:

The basic emotion/mindset associated with the knee is abandonment.

Any knee is gendered: it belongs to George (a male) or Henrietta (a female); on either of them it's a right (associated with male) or left (associated with female) knee.

Every knee also has a front, a back, and two sides.

If Henrietta has injured the inside of her right knee, it's highly likely that she feels or has experienced that a male, or all males, have abandoned her and will again. If the damage is to the outside of the right knee, the suggestion is that she feels discomfort about responsibilities she had, pledges she made, advantages she took, inequalities she believes in—in other words, abandonings she has perpetrated.

If the damage is on the left knee, her gender-related side, then the correlations tend to reflect more upon herself. While injury to the inside of the left knee is associated with believing that a female abandoned her or feeling abandoned by females in general, the outside of the left knee is tied strongly to behaviors of the self, raising questions about all she might not have lived up to in relation to other females, and especially to postures and movement habits denying or ignoring her own needs.

All of this is the same for George's knees, in mirror image. If on the inside of the left knee, the issues likely would be that he has been and will again be, or fears that he will again be, abandoned by females. The outside of the left knee suggests unconscious or unadmitted experience of being the one to abandon females.

If he damages his right knee, remembering that the right side carries the body's manifestation of male principle (his own gender), damage on the inside suggests fear of abandonment by male (Dad). On the outside, the implication is of struggle with accepting responsibility for his own action.

An injury to the front of the knee is frequently accompanied by premonition (remember that the front of anything in the body's map is associated with what is known to the waking self). Injuries to the back of the knee are often a mystery—"I didn't see it coming—it cut me off at the knees." "It felt as though somebody came up from behind and whacked my knees out from under me." Our semantics often reflect what we instinctively know in our bodies to be true!

CHAPTER IV

You Are Designed for Movement

In your physical structure, *position* and *movement* are markers which can indicate the existence in your consciousness of contradictory instructions, intentions, wishes, and behaviors.

At any given moment, the body is charged with profoundly varying responsibilities. If you have a desire ("I want a cookie"), but at the same time you have an inhibiting feeling ("I'm sad or nervous or afraid") and also, as is likely if you live in diet-conscious America today, a restrictive belief ("cookies are not good for me"), then, simultaneously, many physical parts of you are issued incompatible instructions.

The thing to remember is that your body faithfully attempts to carry them *all* out. The arm reaches out to take the cookie to satisfy the desire, but the inhibiting emotion pulls the arm back, and the restrictive belief may stop it altogether. You're likely to hold your arm in a rigid state as a protection against some composite of the instructions, frequently without any observable movement at all—only tension. So the motion is slowed, jerky, and perhaps ultimately altogether left out of your behavior patterns. Grace and fluidity in the fulfilling of desire are sacrificed to the conflicting instructions.

One of the reasons this is true is that no place in your physical structure has only one connecting link. When you lift a shoulder, the muscles in your neck, back, and arm are activated, and with them, to lesser degrees, muscles in your face, hips, and wrists. Not only that, but your muscles and bones (components of the musculoskeletal system) are both attached by connective tissue to the visceral organs, and also sustain them. They encompass and support and define many of the pathways of the fluid vessels as well. So when part of the musculoskeletal system moves or inhibits movement, it draws along with it or inhibits along with it other structural parts of you, and, equally important, it also draws along with it many other nonmusculoskeletal components. That is, whenever any portion of the body becomes rigid, or tense, or bound or inhibited by rules, then many parts of your body, *and many parts of your life*, are also affected.

For example: strict, general, early and repetitive enough instructions against opening your mouth ("don't sit there with your mouth open, flies will get in"; "children should be seen and not heard"; "don't talk with food in your mouth"—everything that inhibits the opening of your mouth) develop neurologic patterning to inhibit opening the mouth freely *at any time.*

Imagine what effect this will have on your entire life! It will interfere with singing, eating, receiving, breathing through the mouth, speaking and kissing. If the mouth is inhibited in opening, then everything that requires opening the mouth is also degraded, not because you made rules against all of those things, but because if you have removed permission, choice, and mobility from that part of the self, from that level of consciousness, all the others are restricted. What's almost worse—more than the movement/behavior's being restricted—*pleasure* in that action is *blocked* if undertaken anyway.

Here's another example. Suppose that when you looked an angry parent in the eye, he became more angry. You learned that you could avoid that anger most quickly by lowering your eyes and slightly submitting the head and neck, a characteristic movement pattern which diminished the intensity you felt whenever anyone expressed powerful emotion (whether or not it was anger or whether or not it was even directed at you). You developed a head carriage, and eventually a whole body posture—a look—that reflected this need to diminish your experience of the other person's strong emotion by means of submitting and avoiding.

Eventually it evolved from placating Dad to "I need to be careful not to upset anybody in the world! I will make myself smaller, in my movements, in my posture and in my energy. I will speak quietly, or not at all). I won't initiate. I will wait for others to choose. I will let other people take precedence. I'll care of others, not myself"—all derived from the overriding instruction to carry your head and direct your eyes in such a way that you don't elicit more negative responses from an angry parent. And by now, other people see you in a certain characteristic style of carriage and expression that strongly influences the way they respond to you—a way that will likely reinforce that pattern for yourself.

Though you originally intended only to avoid Dad's anger, other unimagined and undesirable effects have come to pass. People are less likely to be drawn to you. Promotions pass you by. You aren't chosen for the team. Your younger child self had no intention to make rules about any of those things. You were only seeking any way you could, as a child, to influence an environmental component that was frightening or painful to you. You didn't mean to diminish all those other possibilities. You had no idea your response was even connected to those other aspects of your life.

Lack of conflict within the self is revealed by the grace, ease, and beauty of an individual's movements. You know this intuitively. Just as you can discern when an instrument is in tune or not, when an athlete is "in the zone" or not, or when a room is decorated well, you intuitively feel that the quality of a person's movement and balance signal whether or not, or to what degree, that person is behaving in choice-based—not rule-limited—ways.

How different it would have been if you had found it equally effective to stand very straight, undefended, looking slightly above your father's eyes—at the forehead—so that he didn't feel challenged, but you were still fully present. Your attitude, your posture, your carriage would have changed the way people saw you. Invitations, possibilities, what you expect of yourself, all can change from something this simple.

CHAPTER V

Movement Teams and Planar Relationships

You are designed so that in the absence of judgment and inhibition, emotional charge, or physical disability, many groupings of your body components move as units or teams, often moving together or with others in an opposite path. These combinations of body sites and movement are called *movement teams*.

The term "movement teams" refers to something far more intricate than the mere idea of coordination. It refers to *all the ways that all the involved muscles, bones, tissues, and nerves can accomplish a given movement/behavior with the minimum consumption of resource and expenditure of energy.*

Your nervous system and physical body are designed to be able to do their work together with minimum friction, resistance, or obstruction—to generate optimum qualities of ease, grace, and beauty. You instinctively evaluate a dancer's performance by how little effort it appears the dancer makes. You give the highest marks to effortless and graceful movement. You know instinctively that it reveals not only mechanical skill, well polished by practice, but also lack of internal conflict—the presence of only one dominant motive or intention in the consciousness of the dancer, which is the dance itself. In fact, dancers generally dance in order to get into a state where that is all there is for them to do.

So we might say that when movement is easy, you're in line with or "in congruence with" the way your body is designed, and when movement is difficult, something in you puts you in conflict with or renders you insensitive to the design. In other words, lack of internal struggle makes movement easier; what makes it harder is the personal issue around which you yourself are organized.

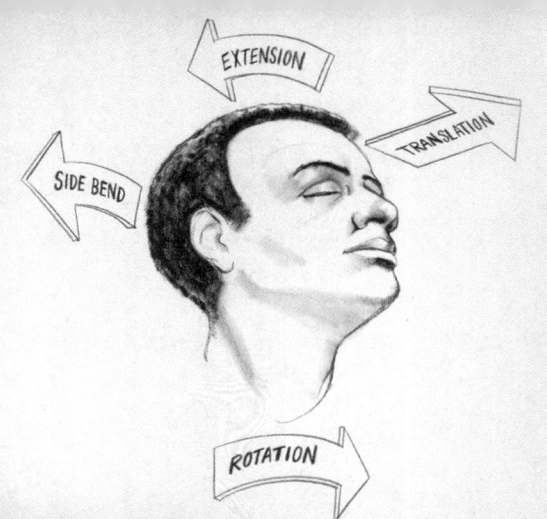

This is a crucial point for the body's map. When there is difficulty, or when teams are moving unaesthetically—out of harmony with their design—then an issue, a set of contradictory instructions, or an obsolete rule is probably waiting to be addressed.

The movement teams are quite elegant, simple en masse, but intricate in individual detail. Some of them involve team members moving *in parallel planes* to support each other's movement, and some teams involve the members moving *in oppositional planes.*

When we speak of "planes," we refer to the fact that by moving through planes in space, any given part of you may be able to

flex and extend (bend forward or back). Nod your head "yes"! It's flexion when your chin goes down, extension when the head goes back. Flexion and extension are correlated with survival, your most basic physical need. The infant's startle reaction is predominantly flexion/extension and is designed to protect it when it is otherwise helpless. Hang your head as if in shame, and notice the degree to which you experience a sense of the need to provide for your own survival.

sidebend (bend to one side or the other). Let one ear drop toward the shoulder on the same side. That's sidebending. Sidebending corresponds with mental body activity, the "taking sides" of discovery (is it this, or is it that?). Bring into your consciousness a recent moment of confusion and let your head surprise you with its movement in response to this confusion. Sidebending is likely to be the largest component. It is highly likely that you nod or twist

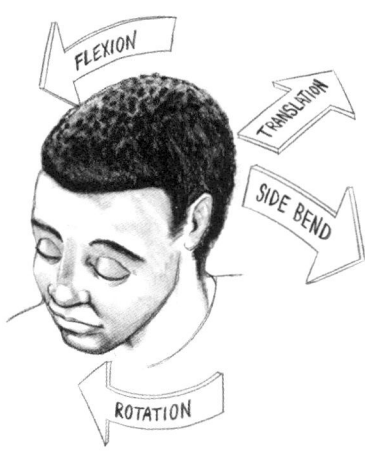

your head far less; you cock it to one side or another.

rotate (turn to one side or the other). From holding your head in a position of level neutrality, turn your nose on a level plane toward one shoulder or the other. Rotation is associated with emotionality. (Direct your head or torso toward that which you want, or away from that which you don't want. In what plane does your head primarily move?)

translate or **shear** (glide forward or back or to one side or the other). Thrust your chin forward while your shoulders and neck stay in the same place, and you will experience this to a degree. Shearing has the effect of diminishing your awareness of that which is just below the shear. With your head in the position just described, what happens to your sense of the connection between your head and the rest of you?

Your head is designed to turn to the side, arch up or dip downward, bend to the side, and shear a little forward or back *all at the same time*. However, if those actions aren't easy, that's a likely indicator that the naturally-occurring teams involved in head movement, on any or all levels of consciousness, have been adversely modified.

TEAMS AND PLANES

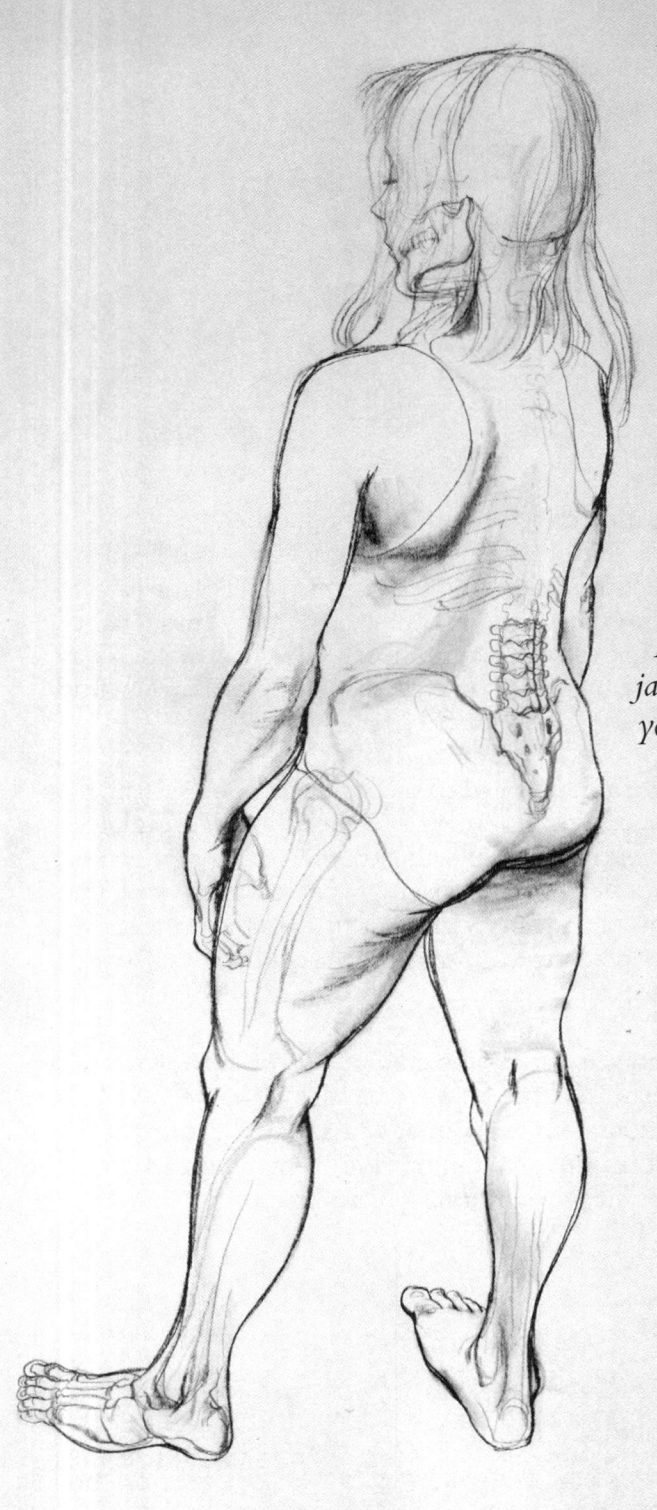

If you tighten your jaw, the movement of your sacrum will also be restricted.

> If you rotate your head to the left, at the same time sidebending to the right and tipping back, you'll experience a certain ease and grace. The whole spine wants to lengthen and the sense of self expands. If you try to rotate to the right while sidebending in the same direction and tipping down, the movement will feel—and look—a little jarring because you are led to compress the spine and shrink the entire self.

When we speak of movement teams, we are speaking of the ways in which specific sets of body parts move together supportively either in the same plane at the same time, or in opposite planes at the same time. Not surprisingly, you can assume equal parallelisms on all levels of consciousness, so that where there are physical movement "teams" there are also parallels for behavior, emotional reactivity, and belief structure/ judgment/mental modeling as well.

Since there are no humans without thoughts, feelings, and physical history—all of which cause variations in movement patterns and the ease of the movement teams—the basic movement teams we are about to describe aren't generally visible in an unblemished state. But we have seen all these patterns in relatively refined states in various individuals, and from them, we can describe an overall composite—not a theoretical ideal, but an ultimate accomplishment for an enlightened being.

Perhaps the easiest movement team to see and experience is the one involving head, eyes, and shoulders. In the absence of rule, judgment, wound, or fear, the orientation of the head in space, the direction of interest of the eyes, and the organization of the shoulders will be parallel, each one actively supporting the other in its task.

The movement of the eyes precedes the ability to move the head (think about it: which weighs more?). There are similar *sequencing* hierarchies for each movement team.

> When you turn your head to the right, what is the most helpful direction in which you can turn your eyes and shoulders to support the ease and grace of the head movement? If you're looking to the left while trying to move your head to the right, do you find yourself more blocked than if you let your

eyes be turned in the same direction? If the shoulders also move in parallel, the movement will be even easier and larger.

The next movement team to discover includes the patterning and movements of the jaw, the relationship between the sacrum and the pelvis, and the organization of the ankle. All of these, too, will, in the absence of contrary instructions, be parallel, and each one supportive of the other.

The free movements of the jaw, the ankle, and the sacroiliac joint are all L-shaped, with an up-and-down, forward-and-back, over-a-ledge glide pattern. These sites are all constructed differently: the jaw floats on a thin sheet of cartilage with muscles to move the jaw forward and up. To move it backward and down, those muscles are relaxed. The ankle and the sacroiliac joint are constructed differently, but the movement pattern is the same, a rocker-shaped L. And the three structures are tied together in consciousness. If you tighten your jaw, the movement of your sacrum will also be restricted (*try it!*). If the ankle is injured, the range of motion of the jaw will be affected as well.

Now, an important point to notice is that this team (jaw, pelvis, and ankle) moves most easily on the same track in the *opposite* direction of the first (eyes, head, and shoulders) in flexion/extension. They *begin* opposite when you rotate your head, neck, shoulders, and eyes, and they prefer to *end* opposite when sidebending.

> When you tilt your head backward in extension, is it easier to hold your jaw closed or to open it? As you sit in a chair and roll your pelvis forward, which way does your head move most easily, forward or back? Sitting with your feet comfortably flat on the floor, when you roll your ankles forward, what happens to the natural movement of your sit bones and skull?

These are general and brief illustrations of the principle of movement teams. (For courageous souls who wish to learn more, advanced teams are presented in Appendix B.) When you are aware of the presence or disorganization of these teams in your own movement patterns, it becomes possible for you to identify blocks, immobilities, and other dysfunctions in *any other* level of your consciousness. Then you can begin to revise them or develop new ones.

Any important rule, intention, or feeling—just about any condition in your life—is made up of contradictory ingredients. For example (insert a familiar activity that makes these sentences accurate for you!): You want to _____, but you shouldn't. You feel that you have to _____, and you can't (you don't have permission, or you fear the consequences). _____ is bad for you, yet you do it anyway.

The result is that the same body parts are simultaneously issued conflicting instructions. You may be attracted to someone beautiful on your right. If you're not comfortable with your attraction, you may let your eyes drift over while you keep your head and body turned away. You may even desperately wish to go up to the person, but actually walk in the other direction. Opposing tasks, or at least discongruent ones, are assigned to components of the body that are designed to work together. So when the planes of movement are contradictory, it is likely that conflicting instructions are in operation.

If the head turns to the left and while doing so sidebends slightly to the right, the range of movement will be extended, it will take less effort, the tissues will be less strained, and the overall quality of the experience will be significantly elevated. If you learned at an early age that a particular movement or set of movements made by one part of your body wasn't entirely acceptable, and you adapted by *rotating* the same part of the body, or a member of the same movement team, to the left while *sidebending* to the left, the movement will have poorer quality, the tissues will contract, the range of motion will diminish, and the overall experience will be conflicted. Yet it may feel normal or familiar to you, because it's such a long habit. The possibility of greater ease in your life seems doubtful because the basic movements are not the easy ones for the body to make.

To apply all this to another familiar example, consider the respected elderly that you know. Everyone secretly (or not so secretly) dreads the gradual shrinkage, instability, and other decreases in movement capacity associated with age. However, nobody gets old in a day. A significant number of the physical aspects of aging are actually the accumulated offspring of long-held adaptive patterns that were incorporated for survival reasons when the person was too young to know the enhanced life quality that could result from making a different choice. Stress or tension, chronic suffering whose origin is no longer clear, depleted energy or repeated unwelcome experience are all associated with the body's continuing and faithful attempts to obey multiple but contradictory instructions.

You can tell when instructions for carrying out well-meant intentions have been misapplied or contradict each other by investigating the postures you habitually employ. You can also learn a great deal about such discongruencies through exploring the patterns of body movements you can and cannot make, and noting the quality of unease, dis-ease, or "ill-at-ease" with which you make them. Having done so, you can choose to change them, and thus allow into your life the ease and effortlessness you were born to enjoy.

CHAPTER VI

Posture

The body's map is not about deciphering the final "meaning" of anything. Like all good maps, it is a means for exploration, discovery, and verification, and can be added to by any honest scout. In the following exploratory activities, let your "seeing" be done not only with your physical eyes, but also with your heart. Peripheral, unfocused, or blurred vision can often give you more useful information than hard staring, if what you want is to uncover the emotions and thought patterns associated with any physical posture. Hard staring is judgmental and projective, and stops true "seeing." Soften as you consider the following aspects of your posture, and let yourself learn.

It's sometimes difficult to see ourselves accurately when beginning this work, so we suggest that you recruit a friend for these activities. Take turns. Sit or stand comfortably either facing each other or together facing a wide mirror (for example, the kind of mirrored sliding closet door often installed in master bedrooms). As one of you (#1, we'll call you) volunteers to be the one observed, the other (#2) will *mirror* you. This mirroring has several benefits. As #1, you get to see yourself from the outside and notice whether you look the way you feel from the inside. As #2, you get to feel from the inside the way you see #1 from the outside. For both of you, this is an opportunity to ask: Is the feeling from the inside faithful to the visible outward posture? What discrepancies are there? This is a little like watching a video of yourself—only better, because there's a friend, and you're doing it for exploratory purposes.

But of course you don't have to "mirror" with a friend. You can observe yourself in a mirror alone. Or you can feel from the inside with heightened awareness. Or you can ask a trusted friend to report to you as accurately as possible the aspects of yourself we will point out in three representative (by no means all-inclusive!) postural-discovery activities below.

Begin by sitting or standing comfortably erect—not unnaturally straight, but in the way you do it habitually. Notice whether your "habit" corresponds more to the way that you sit at ease in front of the TV, or more to the way you sit around a conference table as a valued and responsible member of some committee. If you're standing, does your "habit" correspond more to the way you stand in a line as you wait to get tickets, or more to the way you stand when you're giving a presentation at work or school? None of these is "better" or "worse." It's merely instructive and interesting (and can be highly entertaining, too!) to see which is your habit of choice.

That's it. You don't have to do anything else—except, now, notice (*without changing*) two things:

- the height and position of your shoulders relative to each other, to your ears, and to your spine, and the degree of tightness or relaxation they feel; and
- the angle and direction of the tilt of your head, if any.

It's important *not to change* anything you notice. Just observe it; be aware. If you feel movement or change, become curious as to how and why you're moving or changing. Do you have a judgment in your mind? Now reverse. *Slowly* return to your originally chosen "habitual" position of sitting or standing. Be patient as you consider what data these two aspects can give about the perceptions, behaviors, internal states, values, and (dis)satisfactions you have taken on since infancy. Remember that these are not necessarily the positions you took as a newborn. They may have been developed since infancy. They are your *adult* reality. You *can* see them. Your personality is built upon and expresses itself through them. As such they give you much data about your *current* habits of posture—and the associated other levels of consciousness related to them.

Relative height and position of shoulders.
See if you can answer the following questions as you observe your shoulders in this sitting or standing position—and see if you can correlate both the questions and the answers to the information you have about location, planes of movement, and movement teams in the body's map:

> Is one shoulder higher than the other? Which one? How much higher or lower?
> Is one or both shoulder(s) pressed back, or pulled forward? Which one? How far?
> Is one closer to the center, with a corresponding narrowing of that side of the chest? Which one?
> What other parts of your upper body are involved in this position of the shoulders—the neck? The upper back? The arms? How about the eyes? What else?

- The habitual positions of the shoulders define the degree to which you are willing to have your innermost self seen, and be affected, by the outer world. These positions also influence how and to what degree you affect others. Check internally before you believe this unconditionally. Does this seem true? If you shift the position of your shoulders, do you feel more or less willing to be seen than before? How does your sense of your engagement with others change?

- The more you carry the shoulder elevated toward the ears—the common American form of tension—the more emotional/body memory and mental anticipation of an unpleasant experience, an emotional or mental or physical blow that you do not believe you can prevent. This habitual shoulder position decreases the immediacy with which the threat is felt.

- The more the shoulders are pressed forward, the more shame tends to be involved, because the pressure as both shoulders come forward eventually focuses through the diaphragm to the top of the duodenum, which resonates vibrationally with conscious shame.

- The more the shoulders are pulled back, the more the self is filled with the belief that a) being hurt by others is inevitable but b) it is possible to organize the self so that you don't feel it as deeply. The more the shoulders are pulled down, the more they interfere with movements of the ribs and fingers, rather than expressing the shoulders' own role.

Tilt and direction of head.
See if you can answer the following questions as you observe the position of your head in this sitting or standing position.

Where is your face pointing—straight ahead? Or to one side? Which one?

Is your face pointing toward a point higher than itself, or lower than itself, or neither? How much higher or lower?

Is one ear closer to the shoulder on that side than the other ear is to the shoulder on its side, leaving the other ear further away from the shoulder on that side? Which is true for which side?

When you rotate, flex or extend, or sidebend your head, do you tilt to *open one ear* so that it can receive more than the other? Which one? Or do you tilt to *close down* so that one ear does not have to hear? Which one?

What other parts of you are involved in this position of the head—the neck? The chest? The back muscles or spine? How about the jaw? What else?

- A typical head carriage relies in part upon the occiput (the part of the skull at the rear and the base of the head) resting on the atlas (the vertebra at the top of the spine) and how those interface—whether they move as a unit or independently, and in what ways they move and don't move.

- The habitual positioning of the occiput in relation to the atlas, and the movements habitually made there, have to do with the way you organize yourself to balance support vs. control. The habitual movements and positions of the axis (the second cervical vertebra) are primarily directed by the movements of the eyes and largely stimulating of the emotions. The next vertebra down, C3, is biased toward sidebending and stimulating the growth of the mental body, especially when confused or uncertain.

- The reason the eyes, neck, and shoulders are functionally a team is that your habitual position was patterned to a great degree by two related experiences: a) the touch quality and habitual carriages and positions of maintenance in which you were held as a baby, and b) the way you originally felt from the time you were beginning to develop the ability to raise the head and look around, bringing predominance to the visual field. Both of these are inevitably tied into the cervical curve.

- Compressing the occiput onto the atlas by flexing or extending the head, or by sidebending to left or right, will do something in the chest and all the other vertebrae behind it. Check to see if it's true for you? While continuing to compress, tilt the head back a little. Does anything happen in terms of your judgments or predictions in relation to others. Now, compress the occiput onto the atlas and nod slightly forward. What happens now in terms of your sense of your relation to others? If you slightly tip your head to one side while the occiput/atlas is compressed (sidebending), you functionally compress that side more; what happens to your sense of your relation to that side's gender? This particular set of explorations gives you insight into your own perception of power, support, and control—with the occiput/atlas as both "scout" and "general"!

- The closing of the right ear by tilting the head to the right side goes along with being less willing to take in male reality as you have experienced it. A habitual tilt to the left goes with less willingness for female reality (as you experience it) to be heard. (Check for yourself. Is it true?) Plenty of people organize the head tilt and rotation to the same side because it is a way to shut down a painful charge—a negative association with one gender or the other. For such people, rules are so imperative, or contradictory instructions so

[39]

POSTURE

wounding, that they end up doing everything on that side—they turn their head that way, they tilt their head that way, bear weight on that side, etc. What's true for you?

- In general, how you place your head, with all the attendant patterns, reveals the emotional basis and strategic behaviors you adopted in relation to the right/wrong rules and values that your caregivers had for themselves. The more rigid the right/wrong axis of the parents, the more limited the movements.

Exploring posture and movements can yield specific discoveries which may lead to desirable changes based on your wishes or needs. With experience, you can identify the rules, contradictions, and inhibitions which have held you in thrall; can make changes in habits of tension, tightness, and non-mobility; and can bring more of yourself to be present and available, to yourself and others.

CHAPTER VII

Barriers: Moving—and Not

Exploring movement brings into your awareness more parts of you *as you*, before you learned to adapt to others' notions of "perfect." Such discoveries can decompartmentalize the contradictions you've taken on, allow you to untangle ingrammatic associations, and give opportunities to reinstate your life's original design into your adult choices and behaviors. The result is an increase in the amount of your total self that is consciously active and cooperative with all of your other parts, and with your present environment.

In the smooth flow of things, when muscles contract they produce movement which creates some desired result. When instructions do not interfere with each other, there's fluid movement. You want a cookie, so the muscles of your arm, shoulder, jaw and throat all contract to reach over, pick up the cookie and eat it. However, when the body receives enough conflicting instructions, it produces intersecting and overlapping contractions such that no movement occurs, no joint articulates, no relocation of an organ results, but the muscles are still contracted, compressed, squeezed.

There is a strong correlation between mind, muscles and the instruction to "contract." Since all levels of consciousness are operating continuously at every site, every site is receiving instructions about survival (flexion/extension), about feeling (rotation), and about modeling reality (sidebending) all the time. It is these instructions which may conflict until there are barriers or contractions which produce no movement at all. If Great-aunt Beulah says you shouldn't have that cookie because it's the last one and she wants it, your jaw may get tighter and tighter, but it can't get any more closed than closed!

And there's another dimension to this. Each site receives instructions to contract, rotate, flex, extend, etc. not only at each present moment. It also feels and models and moves (or doesn't move) because of previous experiences and their instructions, and because of imagined or projected needs. For any site, level, and condition, there are differing temporal points of fixation. All the movements associated with strong rules, whether the movements are permitted or prohibited, remain so associated in your system unless you become aware of them and choose to change.

During an IA class, Rondi found that her body seemed to be unable to respond in a satisfying way to any suggestion of shame, grief, or any other feeling. The lack of movement frustrated and upset her. Her teacher suggested, "At some point your emotions have been 'damped down.'" At the time, there was no resolution. As happens frequently in this kind of exploration, something had been started and not finished—she hadn't quite reached the material. The answer revealed itself soon enough.

A few days later, Rondi took a plane flight seated in the rear-most row, the corner of the plane where the seats don't recline because they are backed by the bulkhead. Two young people obviously returning from their honeymoon penned her in, and, she reports, she felt nauseous from the amount of "kissing and licking" going on next to her while the plane waited for takeoff. During the flight, the discomfort mounted, apparently brought on both by feeling immobilized and by the strong emotional scene going on so close by. She remembered the IA teacher's comment about damped-down feelings, and a memory came into her consciousness of her first-grade self sitting at a desk next to Albert, who was crying.

Albert always cried. Somehow as a first-grader Rondi became aware that his mother was very ill, not expected to live, and Rondi cried too, when Albert did. Even when he was moved to the back of the room, out of sight, she still wept right along with him whenever he couldn't contain himself. Finally her first-grade teacher—whom she remembered as tall and stately and aloof—handed her a tissue and said, "Rondi, dear, you really must put an armor on." To reinforce this she wrote the same advice on Rondi's report card, which she found again years later: "Rondi really must learn to shield herself from others' emotions or she will never survive school."

She didn't connect it with anything at the time, but on the plane, frustrated and hemmed in, unable to move in any satisfactory way, she sensed that, being a good little girl raised by two ex-military disciplinarians, she had done as all three authority figures in her life required of her: she had built an armor around herself. Awareness blossomed. Now the armor could be released.

We offer you here a series of instructions for beginning to explore your patterns of movement (and movement denied). Such instructions always include questions and commentary to nudge your explorations along. We recommend that you don't try to carry out the instructions until you've carefully and completely read all the prompts and the commentary. Then follow the steps on page 10 that go with the symbol ⚕. Read each instruction in your own voice into a tape recorder at one-minute intervals. When you're ready, in a quiet, private place, play back the instructions. Close your eyes and go inside to make the observations and movements asked of you. Once you start each segment in the series, it's better to go all the way through, especially the first time. But if you need more than a minute for each instruction, push the "pause" button on your tape recorder.

Here are a few things to remember as you begin to explore your own movement patterns:

- Whether you are exploring with a teacher or by yourself, there is no pre-existing pattern or formula for exploring. It helps to begin with an *intention*. Perhaps you want to alleviate some chronic suffering, relieve a long-standing conflict, or deal with an obsolete belief or judgment. Even if you "just" want to explore and discover whatever's there, articulating that intention for yourself will facilitate the process.

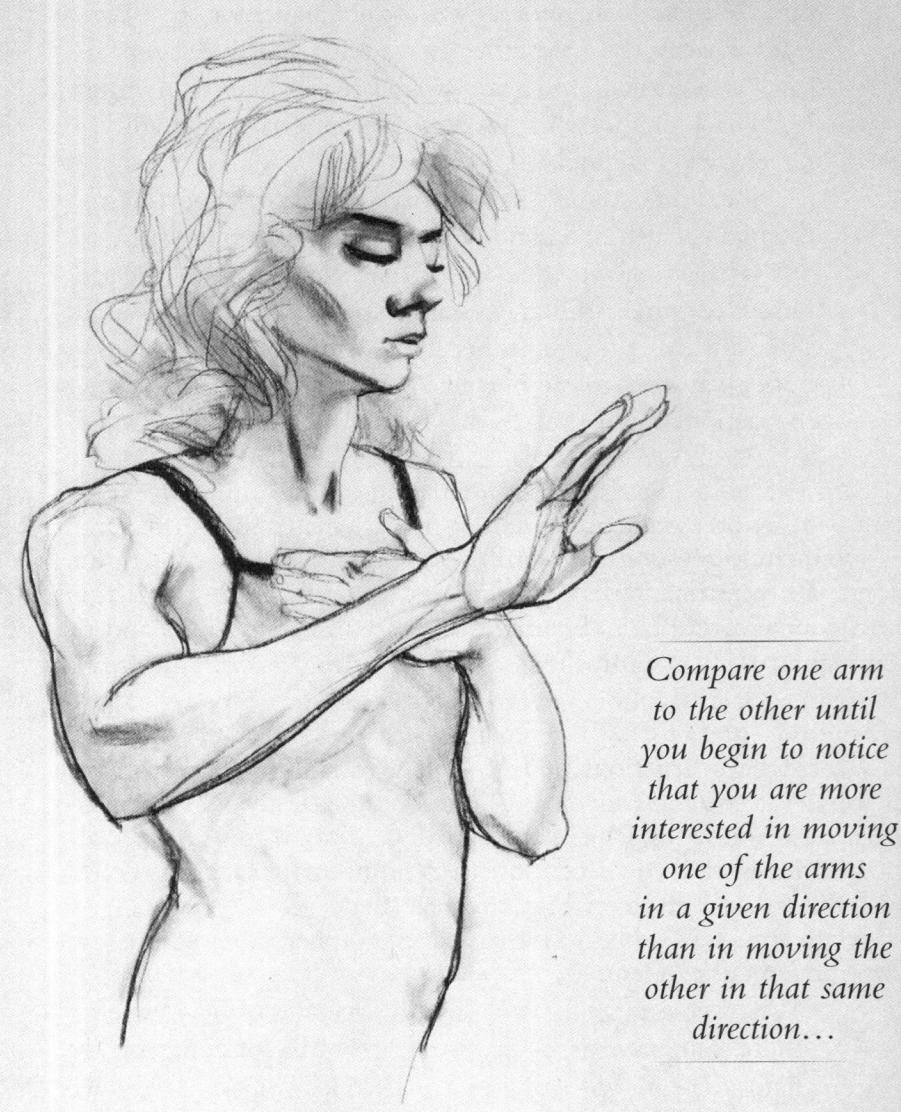

Compare one arm to the other until you begin to notice that you are more interested in moving one of the arms in a given direction than in moving the other in that same direction…

- Very slow movement, extremely gentle and with low effort, will lead to the greatest information flow.

- *Slow* movement also protects you from activity which might take you to the end range of joint or ligament function.

- Gentle movement prevents injury and other consequences of too much force, too much performance (in contrast to real exploration), too little open awareness.

- If you feel compelled to "do it right," if you feel yourself pushing for performance, *stop*. Performance is not the point. Discovery is.

- Whenever you are instructed to *change intentions*, go no further until you notice differences between movements of distinct body parts, or between the movements of the same body part when you change your focus to other levels of consciousness. The range and degree of effort will vary as your intention shifts. Repeat the movement a few times. If you *don't* notice differences, rest or come back later.

- If following any instruction as you understand it, strain or discomfort is experienced where you have had health problems, check first with your health caregiver to make sure it's okay. Integrated Awareness® and the body's map of consciousness are designed *not* to exacerbate problems. However, bringing up more information about a condition can be challenging!

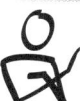

Begin by sitting comfortably, and become aware of the location of one arm without looking at it. Become aware of the location of your other arm without looking at either. Include in this awareness the location of the fingers, the

thumb, the palm, the forearm, all parts of the arm as far as "arm" exists for you.
Compare the two.

Allow yourself to alternately and separately move each arm according to the same instructions below. Remember to move *slowly and gently*, and to *repeat* the movement, *decreasing the effort* each time. Each time, compare one arm to the other until you begin to notice that you are more skilled, more comfortable, more willing and more interested in moving one of the arms in a given direction than in moving the other in that same direction—possibly this pertains to several movements with one arm in a given direction than with the other.

Rotate the arm toward or away from the body.
Lengthen or shorten the arm in relation to the trunk.
Straighten or bend the arm at one of the joints.

Flex or extend the pattern in any way you like...

Add *sidebending* or *rotation* or *any other plane* of movement...

Continue to alternate movements and compare kinesthetic information (movements in regard to position in space which are end-organ mediated) with proprioceptive information (which arises entirely within you).
Notice which positions of either arm bring up thoughts or sensations of safety...of pleasure...of openness... of being closed.

Notice what other body sites tend to go with the arm, against each arm, or don't move at all as the arm moves.

Is there a moment when the movement stops? If so, you've reached a barrier.

Barriers.
Conflict between any parts of yourself creates *barriers*. By definition, a *barrier is the point beyond which a movement cannot be extended or an intention carried out without increasing the effort or modifying the intention*. This is not the same as "contraction without movement." When you encounter a barrier, movement stops until you work harder than you were before to make it continue, or until you change the intention, plane of movement, or level of consciousness. Perhaps when you moved your arm two inches, you noticed that your shoulder stiffened and your wrist tightened, and you could only continue the movement if you used more force. That's a barrier. If you could not even begin to move your arm without changing intentions, associations, or direction, that is contraction without movement.

To present an example from a different body site, imagine that in the presence of someone's intense emotion your head turns easily to the left or right for the first two inches. Then the neck gets tight, the eyes cease to move easily, and the movement in the desired direction and planes can only continue if you use more force. It feels a little like a speed bump in the road, or a scratch on a vinyl record; it's a "glitch" in the smooth running of things. It indicates simultaneous contradictory instructions which may not have been conscious for a long time. As a child you may have received loud and clear instructions from your parents not to appear to pay attention to their fighting, even though you felt responsible for that fighting and urgently wanted to get them to stop. Such contradictions have affected your quality of movement since that behavior became ingrained. Barriers, then, reveal a lack of permission to function fully, with full movement, choice, and learning.

Barriers are not enemies or negatives. There's nothing wrong with them. They represent likely untapped potential, money you didn't know you had in the bank and didn't take into your calculations of what to do in your life because you didn't know about this resource. Like those speed bumps in a residential neighborhood, barriers in your movement patterns are organizational limits you incorporated into your system as you experienced the environment and adapted to it—as you experienced rules *and* attempted to obey contradictory instructions.

However, because their origin is so early in life (95% of your barriers were there by the time you were three), they may not be as appropriate now as they were when they were formed. When you made the rule or took in the information that you shouldn't move in a particular way (do a particular behavior), you were creating safety, or eliciting approval, or otherwise doing the best you could for yourself. However, you're an adult now, and it may be useful to examine the content of the barrier in order to make a different choice and feel more satisfaction or fulfillment or happiness in that area of your life.

Acknowledging barriers invites full range of movement and behavior to return. Without addressing the barrier level, real behavioral change is difficult. If a new movement can't occur or an old one doesn't have the option to rest, it's hard to make a new choice. So a heightened awareness of this quality of your movements can facilitate healing.

To continue from the above movement instructions:

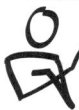 As soon as a prohibition is felt—as soon as you arrive at a barrier—allow yourself to recognize whether or not you know the purpose of this prohibition or what exactly is being prohibited other than "this quality of movement in the present time or in memory of a particular age."

How hard are you working to do this movement?
How much of a struggle is this behavior encompassing?
Do you know what the rule other than "stop" is? Stop what?

If you can't find within yourself the answer to the question about why this movement is stopped but the prohibition remains, whose life are you living?
Whose rules are you following?

You may find that this is plenty of information for now!

Quality of movement is related to quality of life. Deterioration or interference with quality of movement is deterioration or interference with quality of life. Enhance one and you enhance the other. Degrade one and you degrade the other. Notice and decide to change one...and the other will change also.

The bottom line is this: Remove permission, choice, and mobility from any part of the self, from any level of consciousness, and all the others are restricted. Restoring choice in physical movement and behavior leads toward the consistent experience that all the parts of yourself are intrinsically related, allied, interdependent—*integrated!* Without fluid movement, there is less choice-based behavior; without the behavior there is less experience; without the experience, consciousness cannot recognize itself.

CHAPTER VIII

Floor Work

Your body's architecture is not random. As part of the loving and fair design for the earth and its inhabitants, there are consistent, perceptible, measurable signals within the structure, the movement patterns, and the sensory habits of your physical body. In these chapters, you have seen examples and methods by which they provide reliable information about all of the seemingly disconnected aspects of your personal experiences. Your body's map directs you to awareness of the existence in your consciousness of contradictory instructions, intentions, wishes, and behaviors originating and continuing from different ages and times in your life. More complex movement processes, whose designed or unfolding totality we call *floor work*, provide an opportunity to explore and chart those contradictions in such a way that you can then make changes more in keeping with what you want for your life.

Floor work may involve a series of instructions for directed movement which can yield discoveries and lead to desirable changes based on your wishes or needs. No two people on the planet manifest in their structure all the same features, lessons, or aspects, so no two people will respond to the suggestions identically, make exactly coinciding movements, or encounter the same inner-world information. Hence, there is no "right" way to do the movements—only the ways which *you* already *can* (habituals), and which you *discover* (new choices).

With experience, as you do floor work, you can identify barriers to your movements and check the content of the barrier to discover what's holding you back. You can change habits of tension or tightness, non-mobility or non-occupancy—discongruency of structure and energy—and can bring more of yourself to be present and available

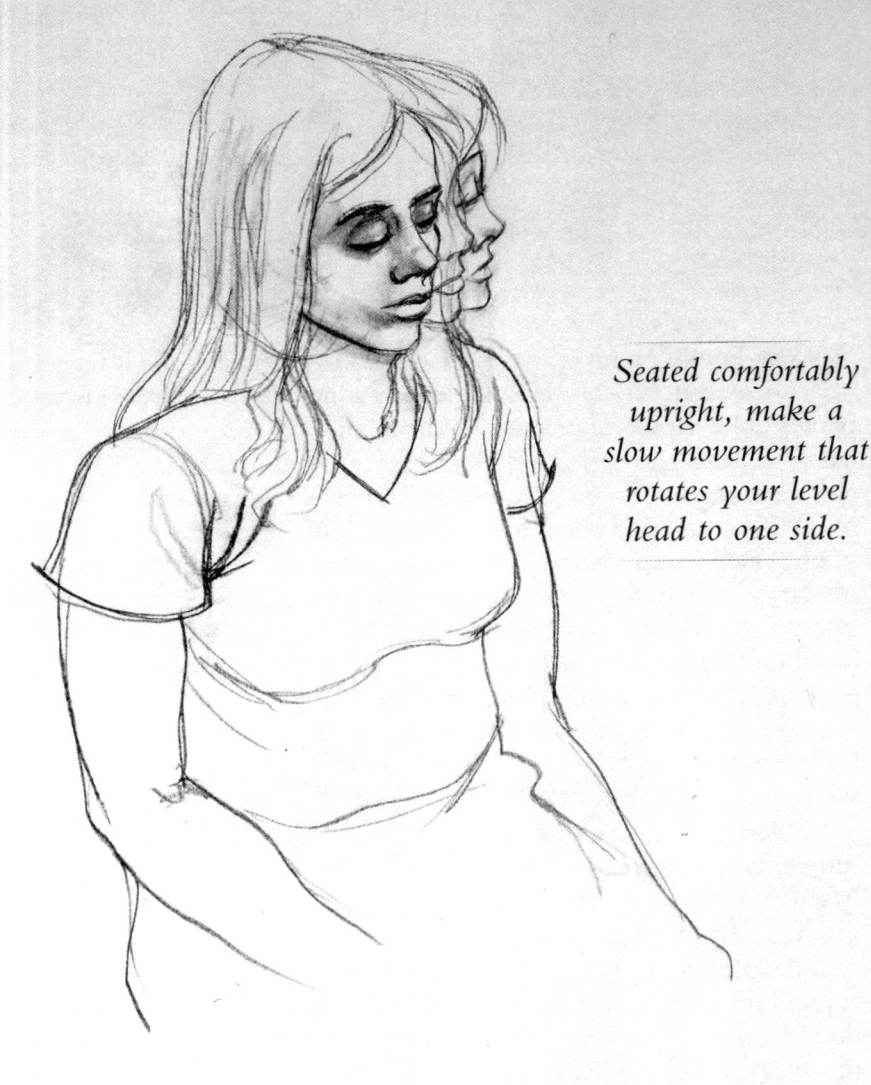

Seated comfortably upright, make a slow movement that rotates your level head to one side.

for yourself and others. And you can discover your own creatively remembered (*not* pre-determined) new patterns of movement, which open up for you more changes in behavior and in life.

You can examine and change the degree to which your movement team members are working as designed. You can dissolve barriers, or turn them into allies. You can work with planar relationships for greater fluidity of movement; and you can heighten your awareness of the various combinations of physical structure and consciousness that come into play as you register various feeling states and human conditions throughout your daily life. In a word, movement processes can allow you to consciously choose the experience of more ease, comfort, and joy.

If it has seemed that up to now in this volume the focus has been primarily on the movement patterns of physical structure, we have done so because it's necessary to start somewhere, and the physical structure is easily observed and felt. But we have also drawn your attention to the relationships between those movement patterns and the emotional and mental levels of consciousness. Those are the ones our society most focuses on. In this chapter, as we progress to more advanced movement processes, we invite you to explore *emotional* patterns through the body's map, just as you do physical ones.

Please review the steps on page 10. Don't forget to leave time afterward for solitude in which to process the personal, revelatory information which may arise during the experience.

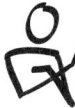 **Discovery and resolution of an emotional barrier.**
Sit comfortably upright, with no bright light in your face and your eyes closed. Make a slow movement that rotates your level head to one side. Turn it as far as you easily can, and bring it back to center.

Turn it again to see if that really is the comfortable limit or if in fact you pushed it too far or didn't let it go as far as it actually comfortably can.

Open your eyes to see where your head is oriented at its comfortable limit turned to one side.

FLOOR WORK

Return to center. Close your eyes; start again and demand of yourself that it take fifteen seconds of continual movement to reach that point.

Repeat this about three times, beginning to search for the barriers.

When you have identified any two, return to center, pause two breaths and decrease the intended range of movement so that it takes you fifteen seconds to reach either the first or the last needle jump or speed bump (barrier). Stop there, and allow your body to choose for you—do not mentally initiate—either the head beginning to drop forward or tip back.

Allow the dropping forward or tipping back to go on till you again encounter a barrier in this second, new direction.

The head is now rotated to a barrier. The eyes are still closed. The head is also nodded forward or tilted back to a second barrier, and the intention to rotate further and tip further remains active and at a constant intensity, so that movement will resume without unnecessary effort if the barrier is diminished.
With the head in that position, begin to move the head in such a way that the ear which is closer to its own shoulder (right ear to right shoulder, left ear to left shoulder) comes a little bit closer. You will now have your head rotated somewhat, nodded forward or back somewhat, and tipped a little bit to one side.

Without moving your head from that position, open your eyes briefly so that you have a visual sense of where your head is in space, and close them again.
Allow the head to choose its own path down toward your feet until at the end, the nose comes to point to somewhere in your torso. Think of your nose, not your eyes, eventually

pointing to somewhere in your torso. If your neck is tight in back, you can assist this process when the head reaches the apparent end of its journey by rounding your spine gently. The recognition of the nose's aim will be clearer.

Raise the hand that matches your own gender (left for women, right for men) and place the palm of the hand directly over whatever site in your torso the nose has come to point to. Allow the hand to contact that location in the way you would soothe a crying child, a comforting touch. Within less than a minute, emotional content, vibrationally matched to those physical tissues, will begin to demand recognition from your personality.

It is quite possible that you will instantly feel sad, afraid, ashamed, angry, frustrated, disappointed, etc. It is also quite possible that you will sense distantly the emotional wave beginning to surface and, out of deep habit, resist allowing it to come up. If you resist the surfacing of your own past emotional scarring, you will likely do so by recruiting a habitual thought. There will be "I can't feel anything," "I don't know what I'm feeling," "this is stupid," "this isn't working for me," etc. As soon as you notice the judgmental thought (and it is certain to be familiar to you, one you hear in your head many times) all you need do to succeed anyway is form in your mind a meaning about yourself implicit in that thought.

"I *can't* feel" means "I'm not permitted to feel" or "I'm afraid to feel," which means you've pointed toward *fear* or *shame*.

"I *don't* feel" means you have pointed toward anger or denial (the gall bladder or the lungs).

"This is stupid" means you believe you are not good enough to do it, which means you are pointed toward disappoint-

FLOOR WORK

ment or unfairness (the spleen), and if it's "this isn't working," "no one can do this," it is likely that you are pointed toward hiding (one of the vertical colon segments) or confusion or desperation (likely to be sigmoid colon).

At any point in time where you believe you can't, don't, or aren't feeling, simply reshape or move your hand slightly or add a second hand to touch the additional place suggested by the above associations, again in the same way you would comfort a frightened child.

Emotional content will continue to surface, as long as you continue to desire that it will. You must actually *intend*, *wish*, to discover what the repressed emotional content is, or you will not. But as long as you do—leaving the head still or to move on its own, *not* by your direction—your awareness will be drawn from the original position found by the head to where that emotional resonance is likely to be strongest. Accept it. Acknowledge it.

In the upcoming chapters we provide many opportunities for you to find ways to make a change in it if you wish. Becoming *aware* of the associations between and among your many levels of consciousness is the beginning of healing.

CHAPTER IX

Defining A Matrix: Your Rules Are Your Patterns

Each body site and level of consciousness in your system has a function that supports your survival and choice-making. On the physical body level, your patella provides an attachment point for tendons and ligaments. The duodenum plays an important role in digestion. Your sinuses have to do with respiration and hearing. In many ways they are independent; each of them has its own resonance with particular emotions and mental constructs, and various kinds of external forces and stresses have acted upon each of them. So they have different degrees of reinforcement, modification and elaboration since their original activation and anchoring.

Nevertheless, when they resonate together in response to the vibration of a specific intense emotional/mental experience, they form a subset of motivations and associations in the body's map called a *matrix*.

A matrix is not an independently existing thing like a femur. Nor does "matrix" refer to a place, like a body site or a spatial component of a body site. It isn't a movement team, although it has as many corresponding components as a movement team. Nor is it a barrier, though it incorporates modified and prohibited movements. All of these things can help identify or compose a matrix, but the matrix itself is a *combination of simultaneously activated sites and levels operating together*.

We have found that there is an "acceptance" matrix as well as a "betrayal" matrix, an "abandonment" matrix as well as a "self/other" matrix, and many other matrices as well. None of these is merely a body site or a movement pattern or an emotional or mental state. It is, instead, *all the levels of consciousness at all the sites that are activated*, regardless of what is also going on at any one site. When you experience an intense and identifiable human condition generally brought on by conflicting instructions—shame, betrayal, abandonment or any of a vast number of other complex human experiences—many parts of you resonate together to create its matrix. Moreover, individual site and feeling components of a matrix were built at different times and ages. A common experience involved with exploration of these patterns is to change apparent ages or to be unclear how old you are!

The benefit of recognizing the elements of the matrices in your system is, first, that when you identify multiple sites and levels activated together in a common vibration, your awareness of the miraculous interrelationships between your consciousness, your physical structure, and your life experience is heightened, and many of your own behaviors begin to make more sense to you. Acceptance—the possibility of choice and change—is literally more within your grasp. Sometimes this heightened awareness by itself can invite change. Sometimes, with your increased understanding, you may choose to de-activate, untangle, or otherwise do something different about that matrix within you, level by level, site by site, as you are willing and able, separately or all at once. A matrix is not a symbol on your body's map to be memorized, or a pathway to be learned, but a set of correlations that may hold a key to your discovering new pathways and possibilities for a life you like better than ever before.

Specific examples follow.

CHAPTER X

Shame and Deliverance

To better illustrate what a matrix is, here we describe two of the most commonly felt and easily traced ones. Shame and acceptance are not opposites. Acceptance *includes* and *embraces* shame. But they *feel* different—almost opposed. Shame is the vibration that, *despite our failings, we should still be allowed to live.* Integrated Awareness does not focus on the morality of any behavior; in the IA model, behaviors are chosen for survival value in the moment, and though they may become habitual, so that they are still chosen even if the circumstances do not warrant them any longer, still, when new or more desired survival options are perceived, different behaviors *can* be embraced. So we do not speak of "bad" or "good" behaviors here. Yet for those of us who have such fundamental self-judgments that we recruit them to give us an excuse for suicide, shame crowds in to plead that we deserve to stay alive.

Shame is anti-ostracism. If you want to survive you must not be ostracized, ostracism being the same as death—"by yourself you won't make it through the next winter, dear." That's why shame is instilled so early. It's very hard to teach a child honor before age four; honor is too intellectual. But shame can be learned from birth, or before.

> Close your eyes and check internally whether this is true for you. If you know you're going to survive a moment that some part of you feels you shouldn't because you're not worthy or adequate, what do you feel?
>
> Alternatively, when you think of a time you were ashamed, what physical sensations, emotional responses, and thoughts arise?

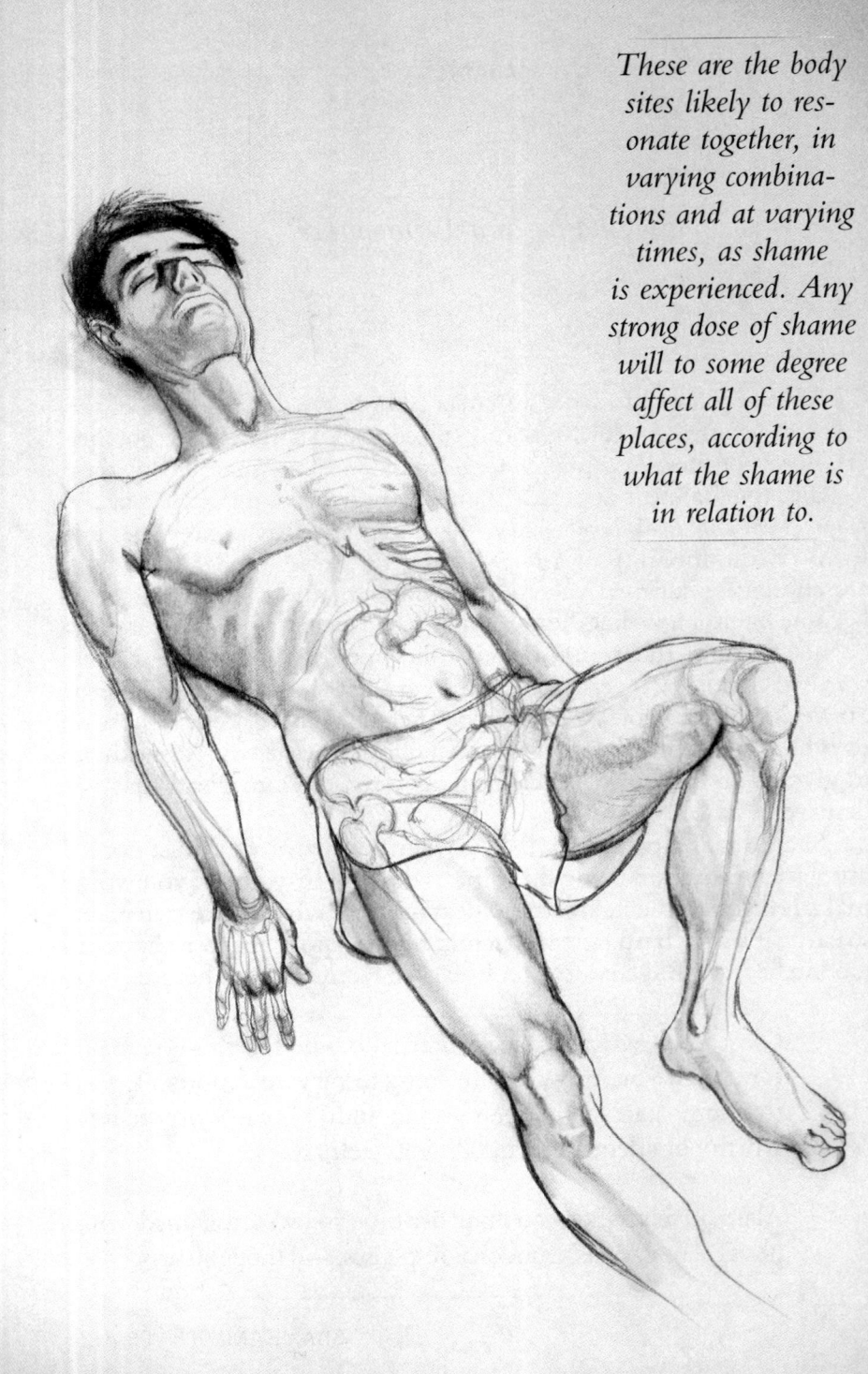

These are the body sites likely to resonate together, in varying combinations and at varying times, as shame is experienced. Any strong dose of shame will to some degree affect all of these places, according to what the shame is in relation to.

On the other hand, it's difficult even to imagine the profundity of the implications associated with a genuine act of acceptance. Integrated Awareness defines "acceptance" as a behavior and a state that many might call "forgiveness." However, the common definition of "forgiveness" retains the sense that something is still wrong, *or it wouldn't have to be forgiven.* Acceptance dissolves the idea that anything is wrong in the first place. Acceptance *includes* the difficulty in your life's journey, delivering you from the need to blame and punish either yourself or others.

> Close your eyes and go inside to briefly explore the difference between acceptance and blame.
>
> Allow your head or your arm to move *for no particular reason*—the intention is to move, slowly, for the sole purpose of discovering what the system will do with a simple intention to move. Notice the directions and planes of movement your body chooses in this "default" movement.
>
> Now make the *same* movement—slowly and gently—while you are *assigning responsibility for one of your life's dissatisfactions.*
>
> How does the movement change? Become compromised? Stop?

Many of us are better at contrition or self-flagellation—shame—than we are at forgiveness or acceptance. We are more familiar with punishment than with the possibility of there being no need for it. Acceptance is a state in which we have voluntarily released any attachment or commitment to maintaining this wound within ourselves. It is a condition in which we can resume creativity and continue our life's work unconditionally. *Fewer barriers constrict us, the further we move toward acceptance.*

As you read about the components of the shame matrix—first the body sites and tissues, then the movements, then some variations on the theme—check in with your own experience of shame and see how it corresponds. As for the acceptance matrix, we will assist you to check whether its components are present within your system at *any* time and, if not, to *find a way to create them!* We invite you to weaken—limit—end if you can—the compartmentalization of your life.

Shame.
First we will describe the *body sites* and *tissues* associated with the human experience of shame. Then we will discuss some of the involved *movements* and *levels of consciousness*. *All are elements of a matrix.*

A matrix is neither linear, causal, nor sequential. Matrices are always associational. Any one, two, or innumerable combinations of matrical sites may be active with shame-associated reality and at any one, two, or several levels of consciousness at any time. Please also remember that no place in yourself, nor any aspect, is ever totally inactive. When it is not processing the emotional context of shame or the mental framework of hierarchy, the duodenum is still busy assisting you to digest your food.

We will discuss body sites from the knee upward.

- The *anchor* of the shame matrix for your waking self in this lifetime is at the patellar tendon.
- The inside of the thigh is highly resonant with shame. (To avoid shame, cross your legs or squeeze the knees together.)
- Two sites that are often active when shame is experienced are the hips for men and ovaries for women.
- The *center* of the shame matrix is the duodenum.
- The pancreas resonates strongly with karmic issues, "original sin," "unto the third and fourth generations" and "the fall."
- *Shame tends to bypass the heart if possible.*
- The matrix includes nerves from the 8th and 9th thoracic vertebrae, and their entire distribution into the body, both viscerally and muscularly.
- The 7th, 8th, and 9th ribs are involved, and the ring fingers—the commitment fingers—are therefore also implicated.

- Either or both lungs tend to be important components in females, and the spleen in males.
- The matrix recruits the fifth and/or sixth cervical vertebrae (the most commonly herniated neck disc), and the cheekbones and sinuses.
- The shame matrix also directly involves the parietal lobes of the brain, close to the coronal suture and the back of the frontal lobes.

These are the body sites likely to resonate together, in varying combinations and at varying times, as shame is experienced. Any strong dose of shame will to some degree affect all of these places, according to what the shame is in relation to. Since each of these places mentioned has other functions besides shame, *what* we are ashamed of, or *why*, or *because of whom* all can influence what sites or movements are activated.

To illustrate the matrix further in terms of multiple levels of consciousness, using what you have learned of the functions in consciousness of the spatial components of the body's map, let us consider briefly two isolated sites—the band of connective tissue that attaches from the patella to the tibia, and the cheekbones.

The patellar tendon is an extension of the coming together of the distal heads of the quadriceps muscle. In terms of your *emotions and judgments* having to do with shame, the more the patellar tendon attaches to the inside (toward the core) of the tibial ridge (the point where you bark your shins), the more you are ashamed of what was done to you. The gender of the person who did something to you over which you're ashamed corresponds to whether it's the right or left attachment. The more it's to the outside of the tibial ridge, the more it's what you feel you have done to others or to yourself.

In terms of social behavior, the cheekbones have a particular function for shame. Close your eyes and recall a moment when somebody pointed out something you did that you did not previously recognize as a mistake, and you felt first embarrassed and then ashamed. The feeling is that the cheekbones melt. They descend and start to swing in. "I'm so cool" does the opposite with the cheekbones. Throughout history in practically every culture on the planet, high cheekbones were seen as essentially aristocratic. In other words, the high-borns didn't feel shamed about themselves, didn't judge themselves; they judged other people—and since we "other people" were all busy judging ourselves, we assumed they were right!

There are also *movement* aspects to any matrix.

An MD friend of ours theorizes that shame produces flexion (the bending-forward or folding–together plane of movement) because it gets you fed. Not everyone in the tribe can be the *alpha,* so how do the non-*alphas* get their share? According to this theory, shame is a survival matrix that allows you to placate the dominant figure by movement (we bow or submit by flexing), constrain yourself energetically and by posture, and displace your desires either spatially or temporally (you scuttle off, away from the fierce alpha, or you stay hungry, don't move, and wait for your opportunity). It allows the less powerful members of the clan to survive by overriding the instinct to get needs met now or here.

Viewing shame through the lens of this "survival enhancement" theory means that flexion/extension movements become prioritized in the nervous system. The most recognizable shameful movement in flexion is bowing the head. Genuflecting is an acknowledgment of the superiority of the other—it's a movement made by a non-*alpha* being to an *alpha,* whether it's kissing rings or altarstones or coattails. It means "I am not as worthy as you, and I acknowledge that." (N.B. It's worthwhile here to mention the difference between shame and humility. True humility does not feel shame, and it does not bow to "higher authorities," but perceives the equality of souls.)

A great many other nuances of the shame matrix exist. Movement planes are recruited for variations on the theme, and we resist or we hide shame with yet more layers of barriers and immobilities.

The thing to remember is that *bodies do the best they can to create a coherent, consistent composite out of incoherent, inconsistent, fragmented instructions!* The physical body is the complete composite and expression of all of your many intentions, conflicting and congruent. What we describe as dis-ease, effort, gracelessness, or lowered health or vitality reveal chronic, noncongruent, even outright conflicting, intentions. If a matrix is all the levels of consciousness at all the sites that get activated when that matrix is lit regardless of what is going on at any one of them separately, there must of course be matrices in the experience of congruent and unifying intentions as well.

Acceptance.
This pattern tends to occur spontaneously when gratitude replaces judgment or resentment, the feeling of being wounded or being excluded, the need to compare the self to others, the fear of intimacy or death.

This state may be unfamiliar to you. It is not a commonly manifested or even frequently seen human state. Nor are we suggesting that by any or all of the processes in this book you will *achieve* acceptance. ("Achieving acceptance" is impossible—a Catch-22—because acceptance is without striving or achievement.) However, your nervous system is absolutely aware of and able to create the necessary conditions. The easiest way to approach acceptance might be to think of it as *aware relaxation* or *receptivity*. We suggest that to whatever degree any painful emotions, negative thoughts, and conflicted habits are decreased or replaced by higher levels of integration and awareness, to that same degree you may sneak up backwards on acceptance.

To give you some of the body markers, begin by assessing the degree to which you already feel the following (from the center):

- Your sacrum and pelvis are free to move in relation to each other, with the pelvis tending to ride high.
- Your ribs and spine do not restrict or compress your visceral organs.
- Your fourth thoracic vertebra is free to move in relation to the third and fifth.
- The heart's actual position in the body cavity turns slightly toward center at the bottom, rises from the top and back of the heart toward the head, and re-establishes a more nearly equal condition of tension within the connective tissues of the thoracic cavity which support and partially enclose it. (If you can trace this, you may be able to sense that the actual degree of physical mobility of the heart increases!)
- There is a resulting physical impression, which can be sensed proprioceptively, that the space between the shoulder blades is widening without the shoulder blades themselves moving at all.
- There is a sense of decompression in the chest where the

ribs attach to the breastbone.
- You may be able to feel that the neck is getting longer in back without the throat shortening in front.
- The rotational movement of your skull around the upward projecting dens of the second cervical vertebra is such that in rotation of the head, neither anterior nor posterior (forward or back) movement of the head is restricted.
- The angle of your lower jaw in relation to the upper, and the angle of interaction between your lower leg and your foot (your ankle), are parallel and unrestricted.
- Lastly, and more general, but blissful and ecstatic in experience, is that if all the above ingredients are combined with weight-bearing through the points of intersection of the arches of the feet, we experience ourselves as weightless, literally as though gravity had ceased to pull us down, and utterly, soul-satisfyingly at home within our bodies, our culture, and on the earth.

The closer you come to acceptance, the closer you come to *experiencing* the present and presumed near-future elements of your life rather than *resenting, resisting,* or *avoiding* them. Resistance is based on the convictions that the injury must reoccur, the hurt will continue, there is no end and no way out. The movements and postures of acceptance, even when only partially present, lead your entire system to be predisposed to a greater variety of life experiences, new and old, because arranging yourself toward the matrix of acceptance restores choice.

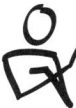
Close your eyes. Sitting comfortably or standing upright, slowly allow your heart to become heavy. You know what this feels like. Carefully observe your internal and neuromuscular arrangement. What do any or all of the body sites with which you have already familiarized yourself find themselves required to change in order for you to move from "comfortably upright" to "heavy-hearted"?

You also know what "light-hearted" feels like. Arrange yourself to feel light-hearted. Make the same observations.

Compare them by returning in an alternating movement from "heavy-hearted" to "light-hearted."

When you have done so, rest for a moment and reflect upon the implications to and for yourself that you can move between "heavy-" and "light-hearted" by intention and choice.

For extra credit (though please, no report is required!), begin from your comfortable upright position and move to "open-hearted." Compare to either or both of the above as your open heart inspires you.

CHAPTER XI

Integrated Awareness

The overarching purpose of the three *Body's Map* volumes is to reveal a more insightful, comfortable grasp of the various levels of consciousness. Then we can acknowledge and work with their interdependence.

The physical body is the essential ingredient of the soul's design for earth life. You cannot do what you are here to do without physical form. We have stated many times in this volume that whatever is physical is never separate from any other level of consciousness. Your physical body, your emotional self, your thinking self, your energetic nature, your movement patterns, the interaction between your soul and the earth—all of these are continuous and simultaneous. What affects one affects all. All the lessons you will ever learn, through any level of consciousness, depend upon your body.

All of the basic emotions (which provide motivation for growth and behavior) are transmitted, generated, recorded, and replayed through the body. The mind is utterly dependent on a physical brain for its existence. Your physical structure is the more earthly, visible form of your energetic nature, and it is the means through which the soul learns whatever it is on earth to experience. Movement or lack thereof, and comfort and ease or lack thereof (suffering), are direct, perceptible signals of the current degree of harmony within yourself and all that's around you.

Just as the physical body can express impaired movement, your emotional nature also experiences fixation and imbalance. If you are "stuck" emotionally, you are likely to be rigid somewhere in your physical structure as well, and if there is chronic immobility in your physical body, it is likely to indicate a similar kind of stopped motion in your emotional awareness.

As you accumulate life experience from infancy onward, you encounter many strange and confusing experiences. You are not born knowing what to do when Mom is sad or Dad is angry, or there's money trouble in the family, or when you move to a new neighborhood and the security of the friends you knew is lost. Any one of a huge list of perfectly normal, *nonhostile* human events will occur in your life's evolution. Because they are unclear or too hurried or you are unwilling for them—because you simultaneously feel fear or dislike or shame or some other "bad" feeling—they become stuck in your emotional self, the same way a fused vertebra or scar tissue becomes unmoving in your physical body.

Thus, instead of experiencing fluidity in the emotional field, instead of being able to move from one feeling to another as the environment suggests, instead of being able to generate new, more evolved or loving or compassionate emotional states, we become fixated—scarred—in our emotional bodies. Our emotional patterns remain as they were at the time the emotionally charged experience was encountered. Our emotional field begins to bend and twist like a river around a rock. This inevitably affects the physical movements we make as well as the functioning of the immune system. The emotional field also generates chemical changes in the brain which determine by inhibition and influence, by habit, what sort of thoughts you are likely to have. And these patterns, being both powerful and *familiar*, tend to replicate themselves in our adult experiences, taking up space and time that might be better used to create or allow in new ones!

The physical and emotional bodies interact but are not the same thing. They each have separate and distinct functions in human life. So, too, does the mind or mental body. The physical body's task is to let you know what is nourishing to you and life-sustaining, and what may be threatening. The role of your emotions is to correlate pleasure and pain, belonging or separateness, love or hate with the physical body's sensations—to connect feeling to sensation. The job of the mind is to *review* actions and reactions *after* the body and the emotional self have created them and then to create a predictive based on the past and individual, even isolated, elements of the present, *and project that model into the future.* So the mind lives mostly in the future. It can be brought to the present moment but it is usually unwilling to do so.

(You can trace the development of the mind in any very young child by the degree to which the focus of the child is not on the present but toward the future.)

The physical body operates always and only in the present moment. You have no way to move your physical body ten seconds into the past or into the future. (Check for yourself: can your hand be anywhere but right here, right now?) The emotional body is *capable* of operating in the present moment, but usually in fact does operate in the past, because that's where the scars in the field are fixated. And the mind, though capable of remembering past feelings as a model or image or concept, is itself without feeling and is oriented largely toward the future. It's supposed to. It's necessary that the mind remember and project into the future the models, postulates, and hypotheses it relates to both physical and emotional experiences. In relation to physical experiences, the mind creates models for *survival*. All of these re-mind-ers and directions are normal mind functions. They're necessary for our physical maintenance and continued existence on the earth.

In relation to emotional history, the mind predicts and projects that, if you behave a certain way, or give off a certain feeling state, people are going to respond to you in a predicted manner. If you dress and walk and move in a certain way, people are going to believe certain things about you. If you violate a "known" rule, behave non-habitually, allow yourself to be seen or your feelings to be known, a previously felt "negative" will be repeated. All these are perfectly conventional mental functionings, still necessary to successful adaptation in a particular family, cultural setting and time.

But the mind has a higher potential as well, which unfortunately is usually corrupted. The higher task is to gather data from all other levels—physical, emotional, energetic—to gather data from every personal experience in order to construct a predictive model concerning the *very nature of our existence* here. From this data the mind's function is to construct a model of what the universe is, what the self is, *why* the self is particularly located here and now, and what the purpose is which unfolds from our choices.

Then, when you move into the next present moment, you can tell, *by the differences* between the elements of the predicted model and what you *actually* experienced, the degree to which your model is not yet complete. The mind's higher purpose is *to find the flaws* in its

INTEGRATED AWARENESS

own model so that it can be gradually expanded and refined until it accurately describes the universe as it is. *The higher mind is nurtured, its purpose furthered, by the discovery that its model is not complete and that there is more to learn.*

The mind is capable of actually enjoying finding that your model of reality is incomplete. If you thought, based on your cousin's opinion and conversation about opera, for example, that opera would be boring and incomprehensible—but then a friend took you to *The Magic Flute* and it wasn't—ideally, you'd say, "my model predicted X, but X isn't exactly what happened. What further information do I need so that the model and the experience correspond more accurately—so that my generalization about this is more in line with how things really are? Where and how can I get that information? What further experience do I need?"

What tends to happen instead is that you might say to yourself something like, "If the prediction based on the model I've been using isn't accurate, I'll be rejected. I won't be able to talk to my cousin about this experience, because if I do, I'll be misunderstood and I won't belong easily to that familiar community any more. So I'd better skew my experience of reality and even skew the data itself. I'd better tell them, and myself, that my experience at the opera really was boring and incomprehensible so that I prove that model to be accurate! And I'd better not give myself any other opportunities to expand my model, because things just won't be the same."

You know from your own experience that this behavior is not a rare thing.

On the other hand, if you embrace that the mind is *designed* for "ah, I haven't got this whole picture yet, there's more for me here," then you can wake up with joy to the truth that *there is more*—more to life—more to *you*—and it has always been there for you to choose to focus on.

The following movement process brings together elements from all the chapters of this book for your exploration in relation to your physical structure and your emotional and mental bodies. It is long and complex. As with all movement processes, we urge you to read it completely through first. Then, if possible, carry it out with the assistance of a teacher, or at least a friend. Allow plenty of time. Each of the three parts may take a whole hour, or a whole afternoon. We present it here to assist you to integrate your developing awareness that your physical, emotional, and mental levels of consciousness are not separate; that, together, in ways you had not imagined, they reflect, maintain, and create your sense of who you are; and that, if you are willing, you can change any aspect of any of them, to invite permanent change in all. You may find that you discover in yourself the matrix for self-worth.

It will take awhile. Explore gently. Be sure to provide safeguards for movement and balance.

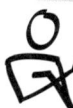

Part I. Exploring "perfect symmetry" and balance in the physical structure

Begin by lying comfortably on your back, arms to side on the litte-finger edge.

Take 30 seconds or a minute in the attempt to arrange your body in a "perfectly" symmetrical pattern. (Symmetry is not perfection. But it is an easily conceived idea of how an outsider might unintentionally lead you away from your own personal intuitive knowledge.) Everything from the exact center of the back of the head down to the soles or the heels is to bear weight as equally "perfectly" as possible, neither tipped up nor down, left or right, side to side.

Change your perception of that basic contact with the floor so that every time you check it feels that you have come closer and closer to symmetry, both sides equally "perfectly" balanced.

Check shoulder blades, and the small of the back, and half a dozen points along the arm.

You want to notice the fingers and the palms and the backs of the hands and the toes and soles or heels of the feet.

Where's your tongue?

What's the difference in openness and closedness of the two sides of your mouth?

INTEGRATED AWARENESS

Don't coerce these changes. Every change you feel it necessary to make indicates an area where your self at rest was not at balance. There would be no need to change if it was already that way. It's important to recognize, though, that not one of the imbalances that made change necessary, as you attempted to comply with the request or suggestion we've made, has anything to do with right or wrong. They have to do with the manner in which you've adapted to the earth! You're engaged in a process of creating yourself to be someone else's idea of "perfect," based on your need as an infant to adapt to the environment in which you found yourself. It's not *your* idea, because you're having to change all these things to come closer. Your idea of "perfect" apparently involves individuality and creativity and differentiation and distinguishing of the self from others because that's how it was when you lay down. For now you're coercing yourself into complying with what you understand our instructions tell you is "perfect"—just as you did as an infant.

Now, if you would normally have any difficulty going from lying to standing, please skip the following instruction. There will be an obvious point at which to resume the process. But if you normally are physically able to go from lying to standing without damage, please hold (like spraying a fixative all over yourself) the exact body pattern that you have (except for changing the bend of the knees) and come to stand—now that you're "perfectly" balanced.

Did the process of getting up while being "perfect" feel comfortable? Is it hard work? Does it feel familiar?

As you stand there restoring the element(s) that you lost in the process of going from reclining to standing in its previous "perfect" symmetrical organization, how's your balance? Take a step.

Take a step with the other foot. In this organization, what are you best prepared to do?

Take another step. What are you most prohibited from doing?

Please return yourself to the floor, still in "perfect" shape. If you skipped the part where you went from lying to standing, this is where you resume the process.
Refine the process again of becoming "perfect"—equal on both sides, symmetrical, balanced. Assume, unless other internal feelings tell you differently, that you have done a good job.

Bring into your awareness any behavior that you *enjoy*—eating, running, reading, talking, singing—any behavior that *you* enjoy.

What portion of this perfect arrangement would you need to give up in order to make that pleasurable behavior possible? This may be determined by retaining your "perfect" arrangement and making the first movement that occurs to you that is a portion of a behavior you enjoy. Stay "perfect" and do something you enjoy!

The difficulty you feel and the need to change what you are/have been told is right or "perfect" or symmetrical or balanced into some imperfect, unbalanced, nonsymmetrical pattern before you can do anything you enjoy is universal. Pleasure is dependent upon permission. Joy and belonging and connectivity are dependent on permission. Further, *whatever restricts permission*, whether you perceive it to be an external command or it eventually proves to be an internal rule, *also restricts pleasure*. Please return to the "perfect" posture.

INTEGRATED AWARENESS

Slowly and gently organize yourself physically as though you were just beginning to engage in a behavior that's fun for you. And it's not that there's nothing pleasurable that can be done lying on your back! Listening to music...watching clouds...or birds...or hearing the sound of children or running water or whispering leaves...

How much do you have to change?

Many people would need to change most of their position—would discover that they cannot be "right" and enjoy themselves at the same time, except by finding some less "right" person to compare themselves to—thin soup, and not very helpful.

Please organize as much of yourself as possible so that you are in as easy a position as possible for the behavior that you enjoy. Keep your eyes closed. Retain that organization (with help if you need it), and please come to stand.
(If you sometimes have trouble coming to stand, carefully use some object near you for support.)

Notice the quality of coming to stand while focusing on the behavior you enjoy instead of trying to be "perfect."

How's your balance? Take a step.

Take a step with the other foot.

Increased permission frequently means suddenly discovering or re-discovering a new or forgotten thing—the way a baby does, since a baby often has more permission for discovery. So your balance may briefly become like a baby's—not so integral, not "perfect," but in an organization of confusion and discovery, with elements of new choice.

A far more important question than "how's your balance" is, *do you like the feeling of this better?* To find out, please restore the perfect symmetrical "you are right" pose in standing. Pay attention to your face, and your chest—especially the heart.

And your knees—is there tension there? How does it compare with the freedom you felt when you were focusing on something you enjoy?

Decrease or cease those muscular efforts which support a particular idea of right or "perfect" without engaging in the other posture (your example of a particular other behavior you enjoy).

If you simply decrease the effort, how do you feel standing?

Whatever you feel unsure of or confused by has within it the potential of discovery. Whatever is so familiar there is no uncertainty offers no learning, change, or opportunity to recruit unknown allies.

Part II. Exploring emotional imbalances.
Please find a reasonably comfortable more or less straight-backed chair to sit in.

In an earlier chapter we suggested that if the dominant movement or postural component is flexion/extension, the lens through which life experience is being viewed at the moment is related to survival. If the dominant component is rotational, that lens is likely to be colored with emotion. If the dominant component is sidebending, the lens is likely to be prescribed for the mind. We suggest that all of these elements and many more—energetics, genetics, time, the component of self that is more than self—are all also present and active. You've just explored a series of arrangements interspersed with movements where the *physical body* was dominant.

Review for a moment in your awareness whether or not there was relatively little sidebending or translation or shearing force involved.

To illustrate the difference between movement for its own sake, movement for survival, and now movement for emotion or feeling, would you please, slowly and gently as you have learned to do, rotate your head in one direction and then the other.

When it's back to center, gently tip it toward the chest and then away.

Let into your mind the possibility that you've forgotten something important.
Hold that as a possibility—that you *need to remember* what it is you forgot—and rotate your head again, comparing the quality of movement.

Notice any preparatory movements you need to make before you can turn the head.

Notice any changes in quality in either direction.

When the head returns to the center position, modify the sensation that there's something you need to remember, which would have the flavor of urgency or survival to it. Instead allow yourself to remember a recent error, something you did that you weren't proud of, which in fact produced a feeling of embarrassment or shame or failure.

To the degree that this is felt as survival-related, the head will tend to move in the flexion-extension, toward-the-chest-and-away direction, probably toward the chest. Before it can get very far, the emotional component, the rotational piece, will come into play also.

Return the head to center and balance yourself.
Allow yourself to turn toward and away from whatever source of embarrassment or shame you've chosen. Leave the head at the first barrier.

Then allow the head to take on an additional plane of movement (flexion) without decreasing the impulse to continue turning the head when it becomes easier.

Notice toward where in your body the combination of eyes, nose, and mouth is focused. If your head is tipped forward you can assume it's on the front side; if tipped back, focus behind yourself.

Is the focus turned toward the shoulder, or someplace in the chest? Is it toward somewhere in the abdomen, somewhere in the pelvis, somewhere outside the body altogether? Where is it organized?

Allow yourself to remain in this position long enough that something (other than boredom or irritation) comes to your awareness as a motive for getting out of this position. What is the "something"?

You have been exploring the quality of movement that occurs for you
  • without consciously pre-associated intention;
  • when you are aware of a possible risk, something urgent you might need to do; and, if you have been willing to come this far,
  • with the sense that you have not done as well as you wished.

Please, now, come up with any justification, excuse, or mitigating factor for why you didn't do as well as you wished.

Whatever you came up with as your modifier – "yes, but…" "it would have been different if…" "if I'd known that…"— notice that the head will tilt more easily toward one shoulder (the ear to the shoulder) than toward the other. You notice this by experimenting with tipping your head each way, slowly enough that you can tell that it goes better one way than the other.

When you've decided which side it tilts most easily toward, leave it there. Call to mind again the feeling of being ashamed, and allow any of the movements associated with that to be added to the tipping…

then bring into your awareness the notion that there was something urgent you forgot, and allow the movements associated with that to reproduce themselves to whatever degree that they do…

So you now have the elements of survival (flexion/extension), an emotionally-driven movement (rotational), and a mentally-prescribed movement (sidebending), all part of the same physical posture. These movements combine into a position—or an attitude. Please leave the head as it is, and, if you possibly can, the shoulders and upper body, and, without risking falling, come to stand.

Please review/repeat, in the standing position, the elements of "perfect"; of "enjoying"; and of this last process that you can recall—or that the physical body will reproduce for you.

Compare the elements of the three different attitudes ("perfect symmetry," "enjoyment," and "avoiding or getting rid of shame") for familiarity. How often is each your choice?

Compare them for effort.

Compare them for relative intensity or difficulty. Is the difficulty more in the physical structure? More emotional? More on the level of mental activity?

Compare them for the degree of confusion, opportunity, or discovery you feel when you focus on them.

IF YOU CHOOSE, REST NOW.

Part III. Exploring the belief in inequality—the mind's decision about imbalance

When you are ready, begin at the position just created, or allow your body to create another, standing, which represents "I'm at risk...I feel embarrassed or ashamed...but I've got a good excuse," all mixed together.

Please take a step, with your eyes still closed. And then another step.
How *old* do you feel?

What is the sense of the *size* of your body?

How *capable* do you feel?

Without letting go of any of the muscular contractions that you can feel in this standing position, without letting go of the contractions—*keep them in place*—override them so that you superimpose your "perfect" symmetrical posture on top of it.

If your neck is tilted, turned and bent forward, keep those contractions, but overriding them, bring your head to center.

If you've done something funny with your hands, fingers, toes, shoulders, or any other part of you, keep the same muscular contractions, and bring yourself to symmetrical and "perfect" again.

Something in this posture, now that you've made the movements to restore "perfection," will feel *familiar*. We assume that it is *not* comfortable. There is a great tendency in humans to confuse the familiar with the comfortable. Remain in this position just a moment longer.

Take a step or two, now that you're a "perfect" person on the outside, but you know that you feel threatened, not-okay, and defensive on the inside.
This is what we mean by "inside" and "outside": The more a movement, a posture, or a behavior is on the surface (outer), or superimposed (imposed at a later time), the more certain it is to have other movements, positions, attitudes, and behaviors underlying it (inside) and conflicting with it. Be honest with yourself: based on having this nearly "perfect" exterior and those other interior qualities of imbalance and shame and inequality, what do you like? How do you judge yourself? How do you assess your value as a person? Just what are you worth?

REST.

The flexion/extension, the nodding forward/back of the body as a whole, and the tension that overrides and lies within it all create an ongoing sense of danger. To most of us, the world appears to operate on a fight-or-flight mechanism not fully justified in most cases by the immediate physical circumstances. The emotional component (in this case, shame) clearly is oriented about something *in the past*, that you've done but not well enough, or *not* done. The mental body, which is habitually oriented toward the future, is engaged in protecting you from something that may happen or will happen again—something punishing or painful or at the very least unwelcome. And if you're old enough to read this book, you have at the minimum tens of thousands of such patterns inherent in your system, learned in the process of adapting to the earth. Similar multi-level matrices exist for all the wounding and difficult emotions—loss, anger, fear, blame, disappointment, betrayal—whatever!

When these habitual contractions are released, however, when choice is restored, there tends to be a spontaneous eruption of other feelings: *excitement* or *connection* or *creativity* or *joy*.

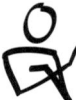 Still holding on to the overlay of symmetrical and "perfect," let go the impulse or contraction that would bring the head forward or back.

> If any movement at all occurred, assume that *every* human may experience at least the same level of conflict within the self that you do.

> Please let go of the rotational component of shame, that either turned you toward or away from something.

> Additionally, let go of the tendency to tip one ear to one shoulder rather than the other so that both the excuse-making and thereby the self-judgment-perpetuating component of the movement are released.

> So now what you have is the same symmetrical posture outwardly that you had before. Please compare it to the last time you stood in an intentional position of balance! Assume that when you did it for its own sake in the beginning, you were secretly following a set of right/wrong rules of your own, adapting to or detouring around emotional barriers. You were accepting the limitations imposed by the presumption of ongoing threat even though it was not in the *conscious* mind. Now you can actually stand in some position that seems to you pretty symmetrical and balanced. In the

absence of so much of that internal conflict, however, it may feel easier.

Finally, let go of the need to stand in a balanced, symmetrical way and opt instead to stand in any comfortable way you choose. How would that be?

Now how *old* do you feel?

How *big* are you?

Make an assessment in the moment: what is your value or self-worth?

Take a step.

Take another step...

The restoration of choice often brings with it the sense of sadness or loss. It will pass. It's the system recognizing the number of moments in life in which this choice was denied. When the system recognizes that choice is now being restored, a different sort of feeling will emerge.

If you've gone this far, please position yourself in any comfortable resting mode you'd like—sitting, lying, supported. Stay with your eyes closed, in internal awareness, for a moment or two. Absorb the implications of discovering contractions of the self (including neuromuscular ones, though it's the self that's contracting), that you were not wishing for in the moment.

How many of them there must be, given the life you've led!

If they were not your masters, how creative or expressive, how dynamic, how much less afraid, of how much more service, could you be?

REST.

We encourage you to repeat individual *portions* of the floor process just completed, rather than going through the *whole* again, because each time you repeat a portion, you will again encounter *more* new information. As soon as you encounter a new bit, cease to follow the directions as you first encountered them and begin the more exalted exploratory process of turning control of the movements over to the body. For a few minutes, allow the body to move and pause as *it* chooses, not because the mind tells you, "oh, let's do this movement," but simply because the body chooses to.

This is a high skill to learn as you explore the body's map. Trusting the self and enhancing self-worth fundamentally equals trusting the body and its relationship to the earth. Things cannot feel okay for you is the world is threatening and you don't belong. Yet if your body is your ally—if you pay attention to the subtleties of its signals, acknowledge their revelations, and allow your system to produce a give-and-take of choice and change based on the data offered by all your levels of consciousness—you may discover that more of your life is available to you, and more astounding to you, than you ever thought possible.

AFTERWORD

If you have come this far, congratulations! You have explored many of the foundations of the complex database within yourself which is the body's map of consciousness. You have carried out at least some movement processes and have discovered for yourself some of the correlations between the physical structure and your emotional and mental bodies. You have investigated what a matrix is and have perhaps discovered the existence of one or more within yourself, as you have increased and integrated your awareness of their multiple sites, origins, and implications. And this is only a beginning.

Appendix A consists of two more movement processes which are adaptable to many kinds of questions and issues that may be influential in your life. You can use these to discover rich and varied aspects of yourself that may have been unknown, forgotten, or ignored till now. Appendix B extends Chapter V by describing more movement teams. There is still more to discover about these and many other components of the body's map, which we explore in later volumes.

Bodyworkers and many health care practitioners have long been aware that touch can have profound effects. A touch can change the quality of a movement (for good or ill) or the reaction response—the experience—at any body site. We have introduced the body's map with this discussion of *movement* because movement can be explored individually and without the charged overtones often present in a situation where touch is employed. Nevertheless, touch has always been part of the Integrated Awareness toolkit, because it allows direct access to neurological and energetic components of the human system. These will be the focus of Volume 2.

To order more copies of this book, or to learn more about Integrated Awareness and the body's map of consciousness, visit our website at www.inawareness.com. There you will find a list of IA teachers throughout the United States who offer individual sessions, classes of many lengths and themes, and support for your exploration. They are familiar with the processes found in these pages (which are being offered to the public for the first time here), and have pledged to help you if you wish. You are invited not only to continue to search on your own, but to join with others in discovery.

APPENDIX A

Two Movement Processes

These movement processes—only two of a potentially infinite number—are designed to assist you to resolve or alter for the better whatever difficulty you are experiencing, and to show you again the potential of the body's map of consciousness for positive change in any aspect of your life. If an IA class is available, take advantage of it to explore these (or similar kinds of floor work) in the company of others. If not, remember to read the instructions all the way through first. Then record them, leaving time wherever there is an extra space in the instructions. When you wish, play the recording back, allowing ample time and a safe space and being gentle as you follow the prompts.

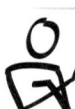

A.1 Finding a Third Choice

You can do this process standing or lying down; try it both ways and see what different data arises. Begin by dividing your body in half. This is easiest (and most fun) if you pretend you have a line drawn down the center of your body, from your crown between your eyes and through your navel so that one leg and one arm constitute the limbs on one side, and the other leg and arm are "the other side." Assume that you can carry different levels of consciousness and different feelings on the two different sides of the body—because you do it all the time, as shown by your asymmetrical physical structure!

Focus on the side corresponding to your own gender (left for female, right for male). Permit that side to make a movement toward an arrangement of itself, or a posture, that represents for you the thing you *resent* or *resist* most about your life currently.

(Variation: let this posture represent one side of any conflict you are currently experiencing—your desire to be well though you have a chronic illness; your longing for a new love though you are still enmeshed with your significant other; your harsh judgment of your child though you know you may have a part in your child's difficulties. These are just a few examples of conflicting sets of intentions that may be plaguing you. Let this side of your body represent one of those sets of intentions. We recommend that you choose only one set of such conflicts to work with at a time!)

Refine the movement and the arrangement by repeating 12-20 times. Keep your focus on the resented, resisted thing, and let your body surprise you with its changing movements and final posture. Take as long as you need to for this—from two to fifteen minutes.

Notice the movement sequencing. What moves first? Then what? And then what?

What moves first is whatever part of you has the most *permission* to move first. It is pertinent to your exploration to note which part is connected somehow to all or most of the related contradictions allowing that part to move. Each new piece that comes in sequence is increasingly conflicted, increasingly less effective as a solution; conflict increases and permission decreases as you go from first movement component to last; later movements are associated with only one or a few of the pertinent contradictory instructions, so they move less easily. What moves last (when movement stops) is what has been forbidden by the body to move in relation to this resisted or resented thing. And what doesn't move at all is, in relation to what you resist or resent, denied, suppressed, forgotten completely.

Notice the barriers. Where do they occur? In what planes of movement? How do you move through them to get to the final posture?

When you achieve the final posture itself, take note of the relation of your body parts to each other, their angles and degree of comfort and mobility.

Hold this posture on this (gender-matched) side of your body. Do not release it.

Now, *on the other side of your body*, permit a movement toward an arrangement or posture that represents for you the thing you *desire* most in your life right now.

(Or, to continue with the variation suggested above, move with your other side toward a posture that represents another potential outcome of the conflict—relief from the physical dis-ease, or an improved personal relationship, or peace of mind regarding your child.)

Again, refine the movement and the arrangement by repeating it a dozen to a score of times. Keep your focus on the desire, and let your body surprise you with its changing movements and final posture. Take as long as you need—from two to fifteen minutes or longer.

Notice, as you did before, the sequencing of the movement, the location and plane of the barriers, your strategy for getting past the barriers, and the relationships of the body parts involved in the final posture.

Take an impression of the two very different sides of your

APPENDIX

body. Become familiar enough with each side that if you were to relax for a moment, you could reconstitute each side. However, keep their arrangements separate and distinct.

Now, without thinking about it or predetermining what will happen, permit your entire body—both sides of it at once—to take on a third position *which feels good to you* and *which includes elements of both sides* as you are now holding them.

Allow that posture to appear.

Hold it for 30-90 seconds.

If you're seeking to *integrate* conflicting parts of yourself *in a way that feels good*, and by so doing bring them to a satisfactory resolution, this movement and this new posture, which *cannot* be forethought, will show you how. When your physical structure experiences that you can simultaneously include both parts of the conflict in a pleasing way within yourself, your entire system finds ways to agree and support you toward a change that embodies that inclusion. Subtle and not-so-subtle changes of perception and possibility will present themselves immediately and in the coming days in such a way that the conflict can recede. Your life can be different because awarenesses and movements have changed, and the levels of consciousness associated with them, not because you "muscled" them into changing (using your mind), but because you have invited the system as a whole—your entire map of consciousness—to create and manifest new choice.

A. 2. Recruiting more parts of yourself

Conflicting instructions can cause barriers, immobility, and constriction. But so can a fixed focus. By being unwilling to include or acknowledge what surrounds or interacts with whatever it is you habitually focus on, you limit awareness of choices. However, your physical structure stubbornly and determinedly reminds you that you not only have shoulders and a neck, but a back and hips and legs and feet. You not only have a head, but also a heart. Your body can be a great friend, as it reminds you that focusing on any one of these things without taking in the existence of the others can cause difficulties that you'd prefer not to have—and that it is not impossible at all to remember and embrace in a new and helpful way that which you have set aside!

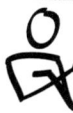
Call into your awareness something that has been absorbing you lately—a business venture, a desire, a failing relationship, a project—anything that you keep returning to, mulling over, analyzing, judging, or wishing for.

Standing or sitting, whichever feels more appropriate and comfortable, allow your body to move into a posture which represents to you this obsession in action.

Take your time. Refine it. Exaggerate it!

Notice carefully the elements of the posture:
- the relationship of the body parts to each other;
- the relative degree of effort from site to site;
- the exaggerated existence of any elements of the body's map you have learned about or discovered so far;
- the body sites and planes of movement most involved.

(You may need some extra time for all of this!)

Now, find an aspect of this posture *you don't like much.* You don't need to analyze why you don't like it—just acknowledge that you don't, and explore the following questions *until you begin to like the posture better* OR *until your sense of obsession changes:*

What has been left out of this aspect of the posture—what body site is completely forgotten when you narrow your focus to this one element?

Recall that forgotten body site to your consciousness. Move it just enough to remind yourself that it exists. (How did you move it? What does that tell you about other things associated with what you have forgotten when you focus only on your obsession?)

What body sites or movement team members are not involved in this element? They're not necessarily forgotten—they're just not used here. Find a way for them to participate. Either move them, or move something related so that they are activated.

What plane(s) of movement have been ignored till now? For example, is an arm flexed, but not rotated? Employ that plane of movement. Continue until you feel something *else* change.

If some of the elements of a matrix are active (that is, highly involved), what is going on with the other elements of that matrix? Find a way to soothe or relax, activate or enliven all the elements of the matrix equally.

What emotion(s) are you feeling?

Allow yourself to sense the manner in which posture is associated with that feeling. Do something with your heart to let the feeling become flavored with gratitude, love, or courage.

What are you thinking? What elements of the posture are activated by these thoughts?

Allow an *opposite* thought to drift into your awareness, even if it seems false or silly or impossible. Entertain it for a while. What happens to the posture?

Continue in this fashion, recruiting aspects of yourself—body sites, movements, levels of consciousness—that were not originally recognized as part of the obsession, until something important changes. You may be surprised at exactly what that is. Not *knowing* what will change—in other words, not predetermining what *must* change—and being willing for an unexpected change that you like, are major components of resolution and healing.

APPENDIX B

Advanced Movement Teams.

For those with the curiosity and determination to explore it, here is a short list of more detailed movement teams. Remember, movement teams are significant in that when members of teams are *not* moving together, there may be contradictory instructions, or issues in the emotional or mental body, which can be addressed to allow greater ease. We strongly urge you to explore these teams with a trained IA teacher as well.

1. The thumb, its same-side collarbone and toe, and the lowest lumbar vertebra prefer to move together in parallel, with the opposite great toe moving opposite parallel.

    > Standing or sitting, press your right thumb against your right forefinger. Now grip the floor with your left great toe. Notice what happens to the pressure of your thumb on your forefinger. Repeat gently until you can feel that each movement strengthens the other!

    > How are you feeling about pressing forward in action?

    > What happens to your desire to move outward into the world?

    > When you pull your left great toe slowly away from the floor, what happens to the pressure of your thumb on your forefinger? How do you feel about your capacity to act? What happens to your desire to close the world out or let the world in?

This movement team's function in consciousness has to do with personal power

2. The index finger on each side is designed to move in parallel with the upper 3 ribs on that side. More specifically, the finger bone closest to the hand proper goes with the first rib, the middle phalange with the second rib, and the distal with the third rib.

With the thumb and forefinger of your left hand, hold the index finger of your right hand and gently rotate, sidebend, and flex/extend that right index finger till you can feel a need for the ribs, head, and torso generally to respond.

Now place the left hand gently on the ribs just under the right shoulder and in the very top right part of the chest, and deliberately move the index finger of the right hand (without the help of your left hand this time) by rotating gently, sidebending, and flexing/extending. Turn your awareness to the ribs under your left hand and notice how they move as you move your index finger.

What thoughts arise?

3. Similarly, the middle finger on the left hand goes with the fourth, fifth, and sixth left ribs, specifically the one closest to the hand with the fourth, the middle with the fifth, and the one farthest with the sixth. The fourth rib happens to be attached to those vertebrae most centrally involved with the heart.

There is a well-known gesture (mudra) of insult involving the specific positioning of the middle finger, and especially the bony part closest to the hand, that produces by parallelism of movement contraction or closure to your heart. In other words, if you wish to curse another person, to intend them ill, since it is difficult to both care about someone and wish them ill at the same time, it's possible (and common) to make a physical movement with your middle finger which is actually a gesture of closing off the seat of caring. (Notice we *don't* suggest you try this!)

4. The ring finger goes with the 7th, 8th, and 9th ribs, and the little finger with the 10th, 11th, and 12th. Try the same movement correlation as suggested above in relation to these fingers and these ribs.

5. The general patterning of movement in the absence of issue or rule is that the hand and foot on the same side of the body like to move opposite.

    Try walking like Frankenstein—letting the left hand go forward with the left leg, and the right hand with the right leg. Now let them swing more naturally. What happens to the shoulders, neck, head, and eyes, if the right arm and hand swing back with the left leg and foot?

6. There are team relationships between the cervical and lumbar vertebrae, and between the lumbars and the toes.

There are seven cervical (C1-7) and five lumbar (L1-5) vertebrae, so we leave C1 and C2, which are profoundly involved with the skull, out of this parallel. Looking at the curves of the spine, the parallels are between C3 and L1, C4 and L2, down to C7 and L5.

> The parallels between the lumbars and the toes:
> L1/little toe
> L2/ring toe
> L3/middle toe
> L4/index toe
> L5/big toe

APPENDIX

There are two of each toe and only one of each lumbar, but each vertebra has both lateral processes and a spinous process. The parallel relationship is between the *lateral process* of the given vertebra and the *outside* of its matching toe, and between the *spinous* process and the *inside* of the matching toe. Thus the *composite* relationship will bear some resemblance to some combination of this; look at the next example.

7. The same parallelisms exist between the middle finger and the middle toe, the ring finger and the ring toe, and the little finger and the little toe.

   Gently move your great toe and then your index toe in various careful, low-force experimental patterns to discover how you can alter the degree of mobility and discomfort you feel in your spine by changing your personal habits of movements made by the other team members also allied with the vertebrae.

   This is especially dramatic if you have a personal history of pain in your lumbar spine. If your fourth lumbar vertebra is held or perhaps even arthritized on the left in the back, then it is very likely that your index toe will begin to stiffen, take a position that is not straight, or begin to take a position from which it does not move as easily as the other toes. Check to see—look down at your toes!

ORDER FORM
Mail with check or money order to
    NoneTooSoon Publishing   or   Touchstone
    893 South McClelland   429 E. Cotati Ave.
    Salt Lake City UT 84102   Cotati, CA 94931
707.795.4399

Please send _____ copies of *The Body's Map of Consciousness Volume 1: Movement* to:
    Name:
    Address:
    City, State, ZIP:
    Phone, fax, or email:

Enclosed find a check or money order for $20 per book + $2.50 s&h.

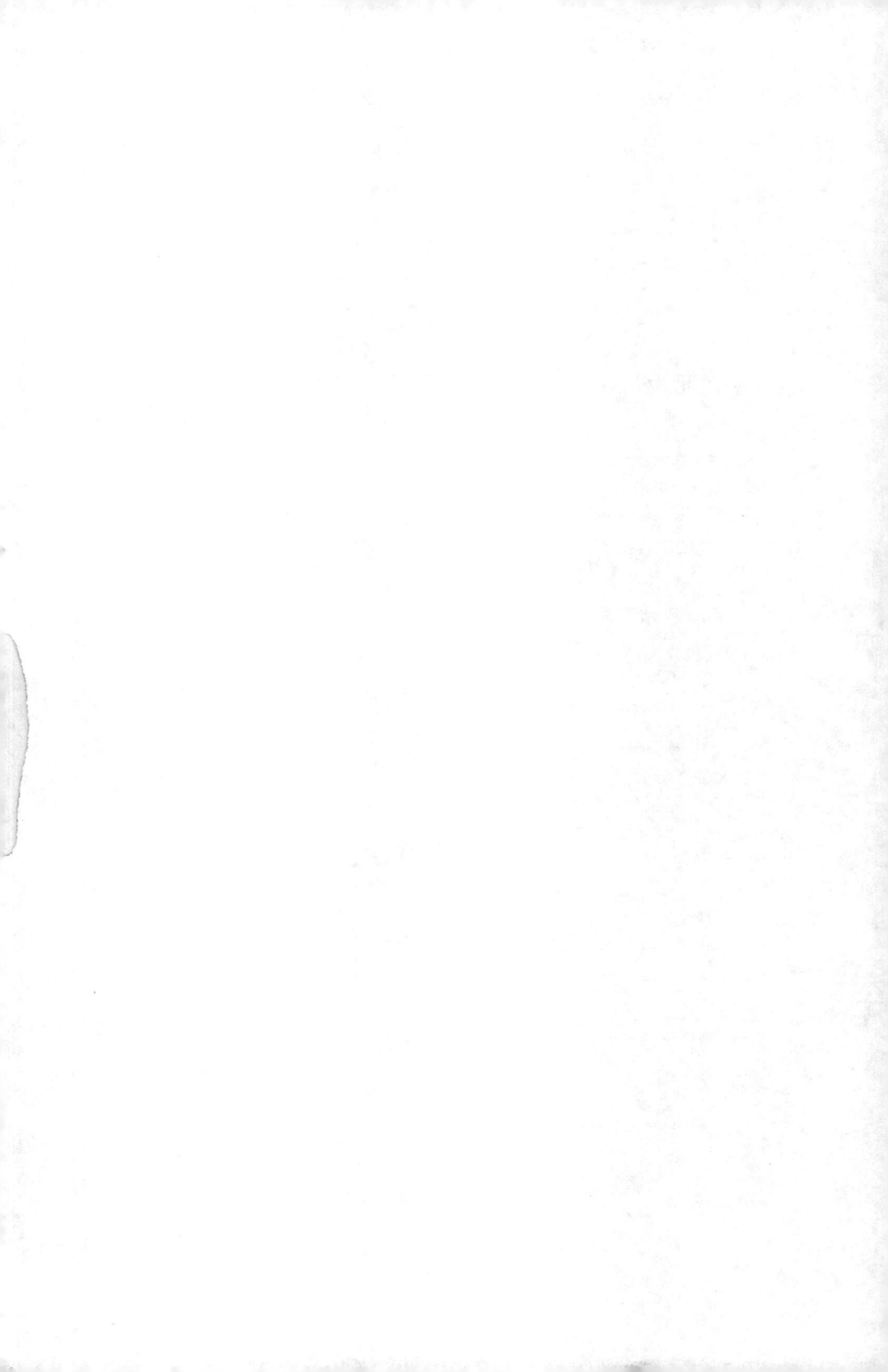